BANISH MIGRAINE MISERY WITH A COMBINATION OF THREE VITAL INGREDIENTS!

Ingredient #1—Magnesium. Discover how this often overlooked mineral, important in regulating blood flow, can have a dramatic effect on migraine sufferers.

Ingredient #2—Riboflavin. This well-known B vitamin has some little-known, supplemental benefits when taken properly in an integrated migraine program.

Ingredient #3—Feverfew. Hailed as a great headache remedy for hundreds of years, this common herb now comes into its own. Learn how it relieves pain—and can possibly prevent migraines altogether!

Find out how Dr. Alexander Mauskop's proven "triple-therapy" program combines these safe, over-the-counter supplements to provide relief from migraine misery in . . .

WHAT YOUR DOCTOR MAY *NOT* TELL YOU ABOUT MIGRAINES

What Your Doctor May *Not* Tell You About™

MIGRAINES

THE BREAKTHROUGH PROGRAM THAT CAN HELP END YOUR PAIN

ALEXANDER MAUSKOP, M.D.,
AND
BARRY FOX, Ph.D.

**WELLNESS
CENTRAL**

NEW YORK   BOSTON

Wellness Central
Hachette Book Group USA
237 Park Avenue
New York, NY 10017

Visit our Web site at www.HachetteBookGroupUSA.com.

Wellness Central is an imprint of Grand Central Publishing.
The Wellness Central name and logo are trademarks of Hachette Book Group USA, Inc.

Printed in the United States of America

First Edition: August 2001
10   9   8   7   6

ISBN 978-0-446-67826-1
Library of Congress Control Number: 2001089375

Cover design by Diane Luger
Book design by Charles A. Sutherland

*To Karen, my wife and life partner, and
our children, Julie and David.*

Acknowledgments

I would like to acknowledge the significant contributions of Drs. Burton and Bella Altura to the research on the role of magnesium. Without their discoveries and collaboration, my research and this book would not have been possible.

Contents

Author's Note

I've been using the full triple therapy I describe in this book since 1997. My patients and I have been pleased with a supplement called MigraHealth™ (also sold as MigraLief®), which contains the amounts of magnesium, riboflavin, and feverfew that I recommend. As far as I know, it's the only product on the market that has the three ingredients in just the right amounts. I've had such success with Migra-Lieve that its makers have asked me to consider being a spokesperson for the product.

Chapter 1

———◄○►———

When You Wish You'd Just Die

I can't stand it anymore! That damned aura, the dizziness, the nausea, the two-by-four slamming inside my head for days at a time!"

"It's the most excruciating pain you can imagine. To say it's like an ice pick jabbing into my brain, or an atom bomb going off in my skull, just doesn't do it justice."

This is how some of my thousands of patients have described their migraine pain to me. Migraineurs suffer from horrible pain that can go on and on. These headaches can become so terrible that some victims actually wish they would die— while others fear they won't.

Over 25 million Americans suffer from migraines. Twenty-five million people crippled by nausea, intolerance of light and sound, sweating, double vision, bright spots before their eyes, numbness and tingling in the face and hands, confused thinking, slurred speech, weakness of the limbs, diarrhea, chills, sometimes auras, and always pain—that horrible pain that never seems to end. Some people consider themselves lucky if the terrible pain vanishes in a mere four hours, for migraines often last ten hours or more. And some throb on for three or four days!

Women are more likely than men to suffer from this terrible type of headache. Indeed, 70 percent of migraine patients are female. Thirty percent of migraineurs suffer their first attack before the age of ten, and the problem is most common among adolescents and young adults. But it can strike at any age, even in infancy. The dollar cost of migraine headaches is tremendous: Over $20 billion a year is spent by sufferers desperate for relief. And the personal cost? It's too high to calculate.

IT'S NOT JUST YOU

Migraine headaches are an ancient problem, dating back thousands of years. Julius Caesar, England's Queen Mary, Thomas Jefferson, and many others whom we've read about in history books were plagued by this mysterious and diabolic head pain.

Countless writers have been victims of the terrible pain, including Virginia Woolf, Lewis Carroll, and Spain's Miguel de Cervantes. Painters are not immune to migraines: Impressionist Claude Monet and postimpressionist Vincent van Gogh suffered, as did Georges Seurat, whose name doctors appropriated when dubbing visual disturbances of the migraine aura the "Seurat effect."

Keeping your brain active is not a shield against migraines. After all, inventor Alexander Graham Bell, German philosopher and poet Friedrich Nietzsche, musical genius Peter Tchaikovsky, and founder of psychoanalysis Sigmund Freud all suffered. Neither is keeping your body active a guarantee of migraine-free living, for athletes are stricken as frequently and severely as couch potatoes. Basketball great Kareem Abdul-Jabbar developed crippling migraines at the age of fourteen. More recently, Denver Broncos star Terrell Davis had to sit out part of a Super Bowl game because of a migraine headache. Baseball greats Dwight Gooden and Jose Canseco have suffered, as has golfer Fred Couples.

Gold records and Grammy awards cannot ward off migraines, or else Elvis Presley, the King of Rock and Roll, would not have been hit with the horrible pain. Neither would singers Carly Simon and Loretta Lynn.

Fame and fortune have not shielded actors Elizabeth Taylor or Whoopi Goldberg. And beauty has certainly not been a medicine for supermodel Elle Macpherson.

In other words, migraines can happen to anyone.

Does this recitation of migraineurs seem long? It's not; it's just the beginning of a list too lengthy to compile. And it doesn't include the most important migraineur of all: you.

IS IT A MIGRAINE?

You would think that defining a headache would be simple: If my head hurts, and it's not because I just bumped it against the wall, it's a headache. If it hurts because I had a lousy day at work, it's a tension headache. If I have light sensitivity, it must be a migraine. Unfortunately, it's not that simple, with doctors identifying numerous types of headaches. And head pain might switch from one type of headache to another, or may meet the criteria for two types of headaches at once!

We generally speak about the four most common types of headaches: migraine, tension-type, cluster, and organic. (We used to divide headaches into vascular and muscle-contraction types. Migraines and cluster headaches were all considered to be vascular headaches. The latest scientific evidence suggests, however, that both vascular and muscle-contraction headaches may be triggered by problems with neurotransmitters in the brain.)

- With migraine headaches, problems with neurotransmitters may be the underlying cause.
- With tension-type headaches, the culprit is thought to be muscle tension, although migraine is also accompanied by tension in scalp muscles. That headache you get after a long, difficult day's work or during an argument with your spouse is most likely a muscle-contraction (tension) headache. Most headaches are tension-type.
- With cluster headaches, the problem may lie in a part of the brain called the hypothalamus, which helps regulate hormones and body rhythms. Or the headaches may be triggered by special receptor sites in the neck arteries that determine how much oxygen and carbon dioxide feed the brain via the blood.
- With organic headaches, the head pain is a symptom of another ailment, such as inflammation around the brain, elevated blood pressure, a buildup of fluid in the brain, or even a brain tumor. Less than 1 percent of headaches are organic, but the underlying problems can be life-threatening, so if you have persistent or unusual headaches, see your physician immediately.

How can you tell which type of headache you have? Only a physician can give a definitive diagnosis, but here are some indications of a migraine. You don't have to have all of these features—two or three is enough to make it a migraine.

- The pain grips one side of your head.
- The pain is moderate to severe.

- The pain is "throbbing" or "penetrating."
- The pain lasts anywhere from a couple of hours to days.
- You may see flashing lights or have other visual disturbances before the headache appears.
- Lights and noise make you feel worse.
- You feel nauseated during your headache and may vomit.
- You feel dizzy.
- You sweat, even though it's not hot.
- You feel chilled.
- You have double vision.
- You have difficulty keeping your thoughts straight.
- Your speech is slurred.
- You feel weak in the arms and legs.
- You have diarrhea.
- Part of your face, or perhaps your arm, tingles and/or goes numb.
- The problem often begins during "down" times—such as weekends and vacations—when you're not feeling stressed.

Just as there are signs suggesting migraines, there are indications that tend to rule them out. For example, if your headache usually strikes while you're laughing hard, exercising, or enjoying sex, it's quite likely an exertion headache. If the pain typically zeroes in on the days you skip meals because you're trying to lose weight, the problem may be due to low blood sugar. If the headache produces dull pain, generally strikes during or after a long or difficult work period, and your shoulders and neck muscles are knotted and stiff, it's probably a tension headache. And if the headaches grow steadily worse over time, they may be due to an organic problem.

We haven't yet determined exactly what causes migraines. But we do know that millions of Americans are susceptible to migraines because they have hair-trigger responses to certain stimuli. Their migraines may be brought on by eating common foods like cheese, bacon, nuts, avocados, chocolate, yeast, spices, hot dogs, corn, or anything fermented, or by drinking red wine, beer, or beverages containing caffeine. But that's not all; skipping meals, stress, fatigue, bright lights, strong odors, certain medications, perfumes or other odors, air pollution, hormonal changes, the weather, seasonal changes, and altitude have all been implicated as migraine triggers. But remember, these triggers only affect certain migraine-prone people. The latest research suggests that most people with migraine headaches have minor genetic abnormalities that make them more susceptible to these headaches. This may be true even for those who have no clear family history of migraines.

In later chapters we'll take an in-depth look at migraines and other types of headaches, their causes and treatments. For now, remember that there are many types of headaches and a great many treatments. Some headaches are mere annoyances; others can make your life miserable. Some headaches can be ignored, while others must be attended to immediately. Some can be handled with a few simple changes in lifestyle or diet; others require more serious measures. Some respond quickly to treatment; others are difficult to deal with. That's why it's vital that you see a physician to get a proper diagnosis. You must know what's wrong before you can begin to attack it.

THE MANY PHASES OF A MIGRAINE

When we think of migraines we typically conjure up pictures of excruciating pain: sledgehammers smashing into the skull or a vise crushing the head. But there's much more to a migraine than simple pain. "If it were only the pain," says forty-two-year-old Nadine, "it would be a blessing. But that's just the beginning of the problem."

Your migraine may begin with the *prodrome,* a period of sensitivity to light, noise, touch, and smell, with mood changes, memory problems, or other symptoms. Then comes the *aura,* the flashing lights and other visual disturbances that herald migraines in perhaps 15 percent of sufferers. Next comes the headache itself, with its terrible pain, often accompanied by nausea, weakness, dizziness, and other problems, and lasting for hours or even days. The headache fades away during the *resolution* period, and you then enter the *postdrome,* the "after-event" phase, in which you feel tired and miserable for up to a day.

Amy, a thirty-two-year-old publishing executive, suffered from frequent migraines. But it wasn't the pain that stopped her from working; she could tolerate a great deal of pain. It was the nausea that came with it that was completely incapacitating. The slightest head movement or any odor—just a whiff of food cooking or the scent of perfume—would cause a wave of intense nausea and often vomiting.

Terry, a forty-year-old television producer, could also tolerate her migraine pain. But not bright light! She had to wear sunglasses indoors, and even then could not go on the set with its bright camera lights. She was frequently forced to go home to sleep off her headache.

WOMEN, TAKE NOTE

A study published in the journal *Neurology* in 1999 looked at the increase in migraines throughout the 1980s.[1] The researchers found that while the number of migraines in men had

[1]*Neurology,* October 22, 1999.

gone up by 34 percent, the increase for women was even greater: 56 percent. And the greatest surge in migraines occurred in women between the ages of twenty and twenty-nine.

Why are women, especially young women, becoming more and more likely to develop migraines? The numbers may be growing simply because women are being diagnosed more often than they were in the past. Or, more likely, women may be hurting more because of increasingly stressful workloads. The 1980s saw more pressure placed on women to work, get ahead, and take care of children, often without the help of a husband. These new stresses may trigger migraines in women who are already susceptible to the disease.

WE'RE NOT SOLVING THE PROBLEM

When the healing arts were in their infancy, dealing with migraines and other headaches was simple: Stone Age doctors used flint tools to cut away pieces of their patients' skulls, opening up the head and allowing the evil spirits, the supposed cause of the problem, to leave the head. But medicine became more complex as time passed, and by about A.D. 800 the British had devised an interesting remedy, a drink made from cow's brain and goat dung, among other things.

Today, doctors have numerous sophisticated drugs for migraines: There's Imitrex, Maxalt, Zomig, Inderal, Depakote, Midrin, Botox, aspirin, ibuprofen, and other drugs. Unfortunately, all these medications can have side effects such as stomach upset, weakness, elevated or low blood pressure, rapid heartbeat, and chest pain. Many of these can be quite troublesome.

For example, I have a patient whose frequent migraines were treated with a tricyclic antidepressant, a type of drug shown to be effective in preventing migraine headaches. However, her former physician did not tell her that this class of medications could also cause weight gain and constipation. Her headaches were under control, but she was extremely unhappy to see her weight rising and find her bowels "locking up."

Another woman came to see me for her headaches, which were partially controlled by propranolol, an FDA-approved migraine medication that is also used to treat high blood pressure. Yet despite taking the drug, she still had some headaches. And when I asked about side effects, she realized that this medicine made her feel out of breath and very tired when she tried to exercise. The irony is that regular aerobic exercise might have been more effective than this drug in preventing her migraines, but she could not exercise because of the drug.

Divalproex sodium is an antiepileptic medication that is also effective in preventing migraine headaches—but sometimes it triggers weight gain and hair loss. One of my patients responded very well to a different antiepileptic drug. However, it caused short-term memory problems that made it impossible for her to function at work. She had to stop taking the drug.

There are newer drugs for migraines, such as Imitrex, Maxalt, and Zomig. These medications certainly have their place, but like all drugs they can cause side effects, such as chest pain, dizziness, somnolence (sleepiness), and nausea. Despite the new drugs, we're still in pain. Twenty-five million Americans still dread the onset of the next migraine, lose time from work, must beg off personal and family chores, and must tell their friends that they can't make it today. The sad truth is that we're still tortured by migraine headaches. We just don't have a drug that can reliably and safely prevent them from striking.

THE "TRIPLE THERAPY," A NEW APPROACH

While there is no 100 percent effective "prevention" drug, there is a way to stop hurting so much: a new, safe, natural, and tremendously effective way to hold migraines at bay. That something new is the "triple therapy" I pioneered at the New York Headache Center, where I've treated thousands of headache patients over the past fifteen years.

Before discovering this therapy I was like other neurologists, routinely prescribing the latest medicines for my migraine patients. I was doing everything right: I was an associate professor of clinical neurology at State University of New York and an attending neurologist at the prestigious Beth Israel Hospital. I directed symposia, wrote papers, and received grants; I was chairman of this and president of that. I had a busy clinic filled with migraine patients who came to see me over and over again. But the fact that those patients kept coming back meant that I wasn't curing them. I was certainly helping them, but I wasn't eliminating their problems once and for all. Taking medicine was simply not a permanent solution to migraines.

Determined to find the answer, I searched through the medical literature, spoke to my colleagues, and talked to my patients, looking for new ideas. One clue led to another, and by the early 1990s I was immersed in the study of the mineral magnesium. Later, I added riboflavin (vitamin B$_2$) and an herb called feverfew to my migraine therapy.

I didn't originate the idea of using these natural substances. Ancient Greek doctors prescribed feverfew to treat inflammation and other ills, while riboflavin has long been known to support good health in several ways. And the first suggestion that magnesium might be linked to migraines appeared in the medical literature way back in 1931. While the concept of using magnesium, riboflavin, and/or feverfew was not new, no one had yet conducted the scientific research that would prove that these three substances taken individually could prevent migraines. Nor had anyone put these three ingredients together to make an even more powerful triple punch. With the help of my colleagues, I did just that. I was gratified by the results, and my patients, many of whom had suffered from debilitating migraines for five, ten, or twenty years, were ecstatic.

With the triple therapy, we finally have a safe and natural way to solve the migraine problem. It doesn't stop headaches in progress, but it can go a long way toward preventing them from striking in the first place. And if they never arrive, you don't have to worry about getting rid of them.

MANY SUCCESS STORIES

Thirty-three-year-old Linda had been plagued by headaches for a dozen years. "It's pretty regular," she said. "There's the terrible, throbbing pain, plus nausea. Light and sound drive me crazy. And even small amounts of physical activity instantly make it worse."

Over the past year, Linda's headaches had become more and more severe. By the time she came to see me, they were occurring every single day.

Although I've seen many people in distress, I was struck by this young woman who wanted so much to feel well again. But was it possible to help her? Her disability score on the MIDAS scale was 35, much worse than the score of 21 that puts one in the severely disabled group. (MIDAS, or the Migraine Disability Assessment Scale, is a brief questionnaire that assesses how much your headaches have interfered with your job, housework, school and family responsibilities, social and leisure activities during the previous three months.) Both stress and menstruation made Linda's headaches worse. She was taking two to four tablets of Fiorinal daily, and she was anxious and fatigued.

My diagnosis was chronic migraine headaches aggravated by the rebound phenomenon due to excessive intake of Fiorinal. I had Linda discontinue the drug and start on MigraHealth™. This is a patented and carefully formulated supplement containing magnesium, feverfew, and riboflavin in the amounts I recommend. Two months later Linda reported success: very few headaches and much less fatigue.

Another patient, thirty-two-year-old Mark, was a salesman for a microbrewery who had suffered through fourteen years of migraine headaches. Striking every two months and lasting twenty-four hours, the headaches were extremely severe. Each was preceded by a visual aura and accompanied by nausea, vomiting, and extreme sensitivity to light and sound. The slightest movement made everything worse, sending shooting pains through his head. After each attack, he felt "washed out" for at least another twenty-four hours.

Mark had used a prescription medication to stop the attacks, with only modest relief. Fortunately, the triple therapy cut in half the number of headaches he suffered—and those he did have were much less severe. A year later, when he stopped taking the magnesium, feverfew, and riboflavin, the number and severity of his headaches increased. But once he restarted the therapy, they eased off markedly.

A third patient, twenty-seven-year-old Dana, had been plagued by frequent migraines since her early teens. They slammed into one side of her head with a throbbing pain that practically immobilized her, and were made worse by light or movement. Sometimes, about thirty minutes before a headache, she would develop a visual aura that obscured her vision. This was a harbinger of disaster to poor Dana, for she knew what would follow.

After a decade and a half of horrendous headaches, and at her wit's end, Dana was convinced that she was condemned to suffer. "Nothing works," she sighed. "I've tried everything, and I still get those damned headaches, sometimes as often as twice a week!"

To Dana's surprise and delight, all but one of her monthly attacks vanished after I started her on the combination of magnesium, feverfew, and riboflavin. And the single headache that did strike responded well to medication. For all practical purposes, her terrible migraines were gone.

And here's what forty-year-old Kurt had to say about his experience with the triple therapy:

I've suffered from migraine headaches since puberty, getting between two and ten a month, each one lasting from a few hours to as long as forty days! I have seen numerous doctors and all kinds of therapists. I've tried biofeedback, meditation and relaxation techniques, eyeglasses, therapeutic massage, physical therapy, chiropractic, acupuncture and acupressure, exercise, dietary changes, orthodontic mouthpieces, herbs and vitamins. I have taken medications including beta-blockers, inhalers, Midrin, Fiorinal, and injections of Demerol and Imitrex, all with varying degrees of success and a lot of different side effects.

When a friend of mine suggested the triple therapy, I was skeptical. I didn't want to get my hopes up just to be disappointed again, so I reserved my judgment for two months. Much to my surprise, the triple therapy made a difference—and a big one! I was migraine-free for those two months! It had been years since I'd enjoyed such freedom from pain. After several months of this therapy, my headaches are rare events. And when I do have them, they are shorter and less intense. It has truly changed my life.

Linda, Mark, Dana, and Kurt are just four of the many people, male and female, young and old, who have been helped by my triple therapy. They're struck by fewer and fewer migraines, and can often use lesser amounts of standard medicine to deal with those that do strike. In most cases, the results are nothing short of amazing. People who have resigned themselves to endless suffering are stunned to find hours, days, weeks, and even months passing without that terrible pain striking! As one patient put it, "I used to have migraines lining up to take a whack at my head. Now they're no-shows, they just don't show up."

So now let's delve into the triple therapy, beginning with a look at what makes our heads hurt in the first place.

Chapter 2

———◄○►———

Anatomy of a Migraine

*H*eadaches pound, smash, and grind; they produce throbbing, burning, and piercing pain; they make us feel as if sledgehammers are bashing away in our brains. And the incredible amount of pain generated by headaches may be even more impressive when you consider that most of what's in your head—your brain—is *not* sensitive to pain.

The brain itself is composed of billions and billions of cells called neurons, each with specific duties. Motor neurons, for example, convey messages about movement from various parts of the body, while sensory neurons handle information about touch, temperature, and other physical feelings. Countless nerves wrap themselves around the brain, and some of these play key roles in headaches. The *trigeminal nerves,* for example, carry pain messages from the scalp, face, and the covering of the brain into the brain itself, while the *cervical nerves* transmit sensations from the neck and back of the head. The trigeminal and cervical nerves carry "pain alerts" from "the outside" into the brain, where they may be interpreted as a problem and then "re-broadcast" as the terrible pain of a migraine or other type of headache. The key point is that it's not the brain itself that's hurting; none of the gray matter is being stretched, twisted, pinched, broken, burned, or otherwise damaged. All that headache pain we fear so much is really on the periphery, in the tissues surrounding or near the brain.

So why does the migraine pain-alarm scream so loudly when something goes wrong near the brain? And what accounts for the other symptoms that often herald or accompany a migraine? The answer is simple: We don't know. We have several ideas and can put together large pieces of the puzzle, but we haven't yet as-sembled the full picture. This much is clear, however: The blood vessels in the head—the "pipes" carrying blood to and from the brain, face, skin, and scalp—are key factors in the migraine equation.

PIPES THAT EXPAND AND CONTRACT

An incredible number of blood vessels, large and small, tunnel through and wrap around the brain. The network begins with bigger arteries, which carry large amounts of fresh, oxygen-rich blood. These branch off into the more numerous but narrower vessels called arterioles, and then into even more plentiful, but relatively tiny, capillaries. The "exchange action" occurs in the capillaries; it's through these thin-walled blood vessels that oxy-gen is transmitted to the body's cells. The blood, now "used" and bereft of its oxygen, continues on through the capillaries into small vessels called venules, then into larger veins and back to the heart and lungs to be oxygenated once again.

The same process occurs in the rest of the body, with blood

running from arteries to arterioles to capillaries, delivering its oxygen, then making the trip back to the heart and lungs through venules and the larger veins. But the network is more than just a bunch of pipes of different sizes. Unlike the pipes in your house, for example, blood vessels are "smart" and active. That is, they become wider or narrower when necessary.

The pipes in your house provide nothing more than simple "in and out" services. One pipe brings water into your house. It branches off into several other pipes that carry water to your kitchen, laundry room, bathroom, and so on. These pipes, like your arteries, carry "fresh" fluid. Once the water has been used, it moves through a series of return pipes back to the single large pipe that carries wastewater out of your house.

This simple arrangement works well in your house because you don't usually demand too much of it at once. That is, rarely will you try to fill the bathtub while simultaneously watering the lawn, running the dishwasher and washing machine, and filling the swimming pool. But what happens if you do decide that you need water at every "station" in your home at the same time? There's only so much water coming into your house at once; only so many gallons per minute can flow through the single pipe that feeds your home water supply. If you try to run the water everywhere at once, water pressure will drop. Relatively little water will come to each station; the tub will take forever to fill, the sprinklers won't shoot water very far out across the lawn, your laundry and dishes won't get very clean.

This will happen because the water supply system in your house is unthinking. It only knows that so many faucets are open, so it sends water to all of them, even if the result is low water pressure and poor delivery everywhere. But that approach can't work in your body, for we can't allow excess demand to cause poor delivery to several body stations at once. If there's too much demand at once, if too many stations are clamoring for blood, the body instantly decides which have the better claims, and which will have to wait their turn.

Let's say, for example, that you're hiking in the mountains. Suddenly you notice that a rather large mountain lion is eyeing his next meal—you. Instantly, several stations in your body demand more blood. The muscles in your legs scream, "We've got to run! Send more blood so we can get the hell out of here!" At the same time, the muscles in your arms are hollering, "More blood, more blood, so we can wrestle with the mountain lion!" And your eyes are shrieking out, "More blood so we can keep sight of the enemy!" Throughout your body, certain stations are ringing the alarm bell, demanding a real big, real fast increase in blood. Meanwhile, other stations continue to ask for the regular amount. And all the while, your stomach is saying, "Hey, I've still got a bunch of breakfast down here to digest, I need blood, too."

Your body, then, has to make some very quick decisions: It sends lots more blood to the muscles needed to fight and run, and to the eyes so they can watch the enemy, and less blood to the stomach, the skin on the face, and so on. Those are good decisions, but how does it all happen so quickly? Your precious red fluid can instantly be rerouted because your blood vessels quickly expand and contract. While the water pipes in your house have a fixed diameter, the "pipes" in your body, the blood vessels, can narrow or widen according to need. When you're running from the mountain lion and your leg muscles need much more blood than normal, the arteries feeding them quickly expand. They get wider so they can handle the increased blood flow, then shrink back down to normal size when you stop running and blood flow returns to normal. Meanwhile, the blood vessels supplying your stomach contract, making themselves narrower. This slows the flow of blood to the stomach. Thanks to the rapid widening and narrowing of blood vessels all over your body, your precious but limited blood is sent to where it's most needed.

The instantaneous widening and narrowing of blood vessels goes on all the time in the body. When it's cold, for example, certain vessels narrow to slow the flow of blood to the fingers. Why? Because the body, fighting to keep itself warm, directs more warm blood to the vital inner organs. Blood sent to the fingers, which aren't essential to survival, runs close to the body surface, to the "outside." There, it cools down and then chills the entire body when it circulates back to the interior. So we only want a minimal flow to the fingers—until the body is warm enough.

If all goes well, we don't even know that our blood vessels are expanding and contracting. We don't consciously control it, we can't see it, we can't feel it. It's only when something goes wrong with the expand-and-contract mechanism that we're aware of a problem—and when it happens in our heads, we're *really* aware of it. It's just this type of problem, we believe, that leads to migraines.

SEVERAL THEORIES OF MIGRAINE

Early healers had a variety of guesses about what causes migraines. Ancient Greeks blamed an evil god, who took up residence in the intestines and produced a fluid that triggered the headaches. Their solution? Induce vomiting to expel the nasty deity.

Some religions felt that headaches were punishment for sin, while Sigmund Freud pointed to repressed emotions. But it was a seventeenth-century English physician, Thomas Willis, who devised what became the basis for the modern theory of migraines: The problem was rooted in the blood vessels of the head rather than the brain itself. We agree today. In fact, we used to classify migraines as a type of vascular (blood vessel) headache. But that's not our only theory of migraine causation; there's also the serotonin theory, the neural theory, and the unifying theory. Let's take a quick look at each.

The Vascular Theory of Migraine

According to vascular theories of headaches, migraines arise when blood vessels in the brain inappropriately contract and expand, squeezing down and releasing at the wrong time. This may begin in the back part of the brain, in an area called the occipital lobe. There, arteries go into spasm. The result is pretty much the same thing you would see if you turned on a hose then stepped on it: The flow would slow, perhaps to a trickle. It's this "slow flow" of blood coming out of the occipital lobe that triggers the visual disturbances some migraineurs feel, for the visual cortex (the part of the brain that interprets what we see) is located in the occipital area. Starved of fresh blood, the visual cortex "throws a fit."

Eventually, the constriction stops and the blood vessels begin to dilate. They become wide, too wide, and their once-solid walls become somewhat permeable, allowing fluid from inside them to leak out into the surrounding areas. Pain receptors in the blood vessels and nearby tissues are set off by the expansion and leakage, shrieking in protest. Quickly noting that something is wrong, the body swings into action. Soon the area is inundated with chemicals that bring about inflammation, causing the pain receptors to howl even louder. And with each beat of the heart, another slug of blood is pumped through the troubled zone, causing another throb of pain.

The real problem, according to the vascular theories, is this "squeeze-release" process of the blood vessels. If we could prevent that from happening, we should be able to head off migraines.

Until recently, the vascular theory held the place of prominence. Today, however, other theories are becoming more popular and vascular changes are seen as being secondary to brain dysfunction.

The Serotonin Theory of Migraine

When nerve cells are stimulated, they release neurotransmitters, special "communication chemicals" that hurry across the gap between one nerve cell and the next. Once they arrive at their destination, the neurotransmitters settle into specific, designated receptor sites and "pass the message" to the second nerve cell.

Serotonin, which is one of these neurotransmitters, helps control mood, pain sensation, sexual behavior, sleep, and other things—including dilation and constriction of the blood vessels. Many researchers feel that problems with serotonin levels in the brain lead to the "squeeze-release" process that triggers migraines. A new type of migraine drug, called triptans, was developed to "turn on" these serotonin receptors and stop the attack.

The Neural Theory of Migraine

The neural theory argues that migraines begin when either certain nerves or an area in the brain stem become irritated for some reason. When this happens, chemicals are released, causing inflammation of the blood vessels, further irritation of the nerves and blood vessels, and pain. One of the substances released with the first irritation is substance P. That's bad news, for substance P helps send pain signals racing up to the brain. A little pain, then, begets a lot more.

The Unifying Theory of Migraine

In an attempt to join otherwise disparate ideas, this theory argues that both vascular and neural influences play important roles in causing migraines. Too much stress triggers changes in the brain, and these in turn cause serotonin to be released, blood vessels to squeeze down, a flooding of substance P and other chemicals, and so forth.

IS MAGNESIUM THE KEY TO "SQUEEZE-RELEASE"?

The serotonin, neural, and unifying theories of migraine are all interesting, but recent studies have pointed us in a new direction. These studies, many of which have been conducted under my direction, suggest that a lack of the mineral magnesium may be the underlying problem in perhaps one-half of all people with migraines. Such people have low levels of magnesium in key areas of the body. And without that precious mineral, serotonin levels are not properly regulated, blood vessels don't retain their proper size, inflammation sets in, and you're on your way to a migraine. Magnesium not only helps regulate blood vessel size, it also helps them respond to other chemicals in the body that keep them from squeezing or releasing inappropriately. So a lack of magnesium can be a double or triple whammy.

The magnesium-depletion theory makes good biochemical sense. But does it go on to the next step? Does it offer us a way to stop migraines? The answer is yes. I've used magnesium injections and supplements to help many migraine patients. Depending on the patient and whether or not the magnesium is given via injection or supplement, this mineral can stop migraines in their tracks, reduce their severity, cut way back on the number of new migraines, and/or eliminate them almost entirely. For millions and millions of people, magnesium is the key to stopping the migraine-inducing squeeze-release process. (I'll go into greater detail about my magnesium/migraine discoveries in chapters 3 and 4.)

THE FIVE PHASES OF MIGRAINE

Whether caused by a lack of magnesium, serotonin imbalances, electrical changes in the brain, or stress, migraines hurt. And the pain may be just the beginning of the problem, for migraine headaches are part of a larger syndrome. Migraines are much more than a pain in the head: They're a whole-body problem.

In about 80 percent of migraineurs, the process begins with the prodrome, or warning phase. Hours, or even a full day before the pain arrives, you begin to feel "off." Perhaps you're moody and depressed, or euphoric and unusually energized. Maybe you're tired or drowsy; you might yawn a lot. You may not be able to concentrate well or remember things you should. You might have a craving for certain foods, like sweets, or not have much of an appetite at all. Sound, light, and/or touch may be very annoying, even painful. Your eyes may become teary, your nose stuffy and runny. Your neck and shoulders may be stiff and you may have some trouble speaking. You get a vague feeling that something has gone wrong; you might recognize this as the beginning of a migraine.

Jennifer always knew that the days when she found herself super-energetic, highly productive, and very happy were days that preceded a major migraine. It was great to feel so energized and joyful, until she realized what was to come. Sarah had a different kind of warning. She knew that if the day began with a sense of anxiety, plus tightness in her neck and shoulders, she would have a severe migraine attack and be forced to leave work early. The good news is that if you learn to recognize the symptoms of your prodrome, you can prepare for what's coming.

For some 15 percent of migraine sufferers, the next step is the aura. Lasting for several minutes, perhaps as long as an hour, the aura phase is characterized by strange visual images. You may see a hazy light, stars, spots, or lines that aren't there, or perhaps splashes of color or vague, poorly formed images. Everything may seem to flicker or sparkle or shimmer, or maybe you just don't see well at all. Things may look white or grayish, or there might be a dark spot (blank area) in your field of vision. Surrounding that blank area may be flickering, sparkling, or shimmering light. Only a small minority of migraineurs has migraines with aura, or what we used to refer to as a *classic migraine.* Most have migraines without aura, or what we used to call *common migraines.*

Next comes the headache itself, that terrible pain. For a couple of hours or a couple of days, your head is gripped by that pounding, pulsating, throbbing, or gripping pain. It's been described as "a nail being driven into my skull," "a wrecking ball slamming into my head over and over," "an endless series of explosions," and "pure hell." The pain typically grips one side of the head, although it may switch sides from headache to headache, and sometimes the attack involves the entire head at once.

I myself have occasional migraines, but I have never had very severe pain (although the nausea is most incapacitating). I used to be skeptical when people would tell me, "I would rather be dead than have a migraine." However, after hearing this exact expression from many patients, I have come to understand how intense this pain can be.

Unfortunately, for many the pain is just the beginning. There's also nausea, vomiting, and perhaps diarrhea. Sound and light can make everything seem worse, so you may just want to curl up in a dark room, stick some plugs in your ears, lay a cool cloth over your forehead, and not move. You may lose your appetite, and the muscles in your neck and head may be sore. You may feel cold all over; perhaps your hands and feet will turn bluish. Part of your face or arm may tingle and/or feel numb. Unfortunately, you don't just hurt; you feel sick and miserable as well. And in some people it's even worse, with dizziness, rapid heartbeat, sweating, and feelings of faintness.

Finally, hours or even days after it began, the pain starts to fade away. This is the resolution phase: Your head doesn't hurt anymore but you still don't feel good. You're exhausted, perhaps depressed, and still nauseous. Your scalp feels sore. You might feel like you're back in the warning phase, with that "off" feeling. Or maybe you're so relieved to be free of the pain that you feel euphoric.

The resolution phase doesn't occur in everyone. Sometimes your head just stops pounding and that's the end of that.

OTHER MIGRAINE TYPES

When we speak of migraines, we usually mean either migraine with aura or migraine without aura. But there are other rare types:

- *Basilar migraine,* characterized by dizziness, faintness, double vision, and poor coordination.
- *Hemiplegic migraine,* notable because sufferers have trouble

moving one side of the body during, and often for a time after, an attack.

- *Ophthalmoplegic migraine,* with symptoms centering on the eyes. When it strikes, you may be unable to move your eyes properly and you might suffer from double vision.
- *Retinal migraine,* with a darkening of or complete loss of vision, usually in one eye.

Then there's the "menstrual migraine," which hits during specific times of a woman's monthly cycle. Some 70 percent of women report that their migraines strike just before, during, or just after their monthly periods. In over half of female migraineurs, the problem has been linked to fluctuating hormones, most likely estrogen. For most people an excess of estrogen probably isn't the cause of migraines, otherwise pregnant women in their second and third trimesters, with their high estrogen levels, would have many migraines, yet they typically do not. A lack of estrogen isn't usually the problem, either, for women tend to have fewer migraines in their old age, when estrogen levels fall off. Most likely, the problem is the sudden drop in estrogen levels during the four or five days preceding menstruation.

A SPECIAL NOTE ON SINUS HEADACHES

Migraines can be confused with—and mistakenly diagnosed as—sinus headaches because the migraine pain may happen to be in the area of the sinuses. Sinus headaches—pain centering in the sinuses, possibly accompanied by fever and other symptoms—are a fairly common malady. There are two types of sinus headaches, acute and chronic, both due to an inflammation of the sinus cavities called *sinusitis.*

With acute sinus headaches, the inflammation is caused by an infection. This can be a serious problem, for the "germ" that triggered the infection and inflammation can slip over to the brain and cause serious trouble. Tenderness in the sinus area, plus fever, headache, and a greenish yellow discharge from the throat or nose, are symptoms of acute sinus headaches. There may also be dizziness and nausea.

Chronic sinus headaches are also caused by inflammation, but there may be no infection. You might feel headache pain, or a feeling of "stuffiness" or "fullness" instead of pain. Moving your head makes the pain or stuffiness worse. A fever is usually not present.

If it's a sinus headache, you can expect to see a stuffy or runny nose. But don't be misled by the fact that you get relief from a decongestant, such as Tylenol Sinus or pseudoephedrine (Sudafed), for migraine headaches sometimes respond to such medications.

MIGRAINE TRIGGERS, GENES, AND THRESHOLD

Sudden changes in estrogen levels are not the only things that might trigger a migraine. For reasons we don't fully understand, there's a host of potential migraine triggers, ranging from alcohol to cigarette smoke, from emotional stress to aged cheese. (We'll examine the migraine triggers closely in chapter 6.)

It's very clear that certain migraine triggers kick off the "big event" in millions and millions of people—but leave tens of millions more untouched. But why does eating a banana turn one person's head into a "miniature nuclear war," yet leave the rest of us untouched? Why do certain perfumes send some people to bed for three days with overwhelming pain and nausea, and make others think of romance?

We know that various migraine triggers affect some people but not others. We also know that half of all migraineurs have at least one close relative who also suffers from these headaches. These two observations have led researchers to speculate about a "migraine gene" that might be passed down through the generations. We haven't yet found that migraine gene or set of genes, except in an uncommon form of migraine called *familial hemiplegic migraine.* (This type of migraine causes a paralysis of one side of the body that can precede, and then outlast, the actual headache by hours and sometimes days.) But most migraineurs do seem to inherit a predisposition to the syndrome. In other words, they're more likely than others to suffer, but won't get a migraine unless some other condition is met—that is, unless they encounter a trigger that sets everything in motion.

Sometimes the trigger is obvious; other times it's terribly hard to find. For example, being under a lot of stress will routinely trigger migraines in susceptible people. But oddly enough, these headaches often strike on weekends or other "down times" when stress levels are lower. So being stressed out may not, by itself, be enough to trigger a migraine.

Could it be that the sudden lack of stress, like a sudden fall in estrogen levels, triggers the migraine? We just don't know. But you'll learn how to identify potential triggers in chapter 6, and how to avoid them.

Children and Migraines

Migraines aren't just for grown-ups. Young children, even infants, can be stricken with this terrible head pain.

Some 85 percent of child migraineurs have migraines without aura; the rest have migraines with aura.

Migraines in children may be similar to those that strike adults, or may differ. Children might have pain on both sides of the head, rather than on only one side. And the duration of the pain may be relatively brief, perhaps only a few hours or less. In addition, youngsters may suffer from nausea, sensitivity to light, sound, and strong odors, and other symptoms. Young girls, especially, are prone to dizziness during migraines. Many children vomit 30–60 minutes after the migraine begins. And sometimes children have "pain-free" migraines: They're struck by some of the other symptoms associated with migraines, but not the head pain itself.

Like adults, many children will want nothing more than to lie down in a quiet, dark room during the attack, hoping to go to sleep and wake up without the pain. Between attacks, the young migraineurs appear to be completely normal.

Because both sides of the head may hurt and the pain may only last a few hours—or they may have no head pain at all—migraines in children sometimes go unrecognized, even by physicians.

WHEN IS A HEADACHE *NOT* A MIGRAINE?

We don't have a definitive test for migraines. We can't simply measure something in the blood or take an X ray and say, "Ah-ha!" Instead, the diagnosis has to be made on the basis of both symptoms and family history.

Not every head pain is a migraine, of course. There are tension headaches, cluster headaches, organic headaches, and others. Here are some lists of symptoms commonly seen in other types of headaches:

You May Have Cluster Headaches If . . .

- The headaches come in groups—one or several per day over many days, weeks, or months.
- The headache typically lasts between 30 and 90 minutes.
- The pain starts in the upper part of one side of the head or face.
- The pain is mild in the beginning, but quickly escalates to excruciating.
- The pain can be described as "burning," "piercing," "boring," or "throbbing."
- The headache seems to emanate from behind the eye on the affected side of the face.
- That eye becomes teary, possibly bloodshot, and droopy.
- The nostril on the pained side of the face runs or becomes congested.
- There is sweating or flushing on the pained side of the face.
- The pain and other problems stay on one side of the head (although they can switch sides).
- Pacing, rocking, and even hitting the head is preferable to lying still.

Cluster headaches are similar to migraines in that they're caused by disturbances of the blood vessels in the head. But the underlying cause is different, and the most common victims, by far, are men ages twenty to forty. (Women are the main targets of migraines.) The clustering of attacks (one or several per day for days, weeks, or months) is another clue to their type.

You May Have Tension-Type Headaches If . . .

- The pain is mild to moderate.
- The pain is steady, not throbbing or jabbing.
- The pain can be described as a dull ache.
- It feels like there is a band of pressure on the upper part of the head, like a too-tight hat or headband.
- The pain affects both sides of the head.
- The pain comes on bit by bit, rather than hitting all at once, and later fades away rather than disappearing all at once.
- The headache often begins some time during sleep.
- It strikes during times of stress.
- The neck and shoulder muscles are tense and possibly tender.
- There is no special sensitivity to light, sound, or movement.
- There is no nausea.
- There are no visual disturbances before the headache begins.

Ninety percent of the headaches that strike most of us day in and day out are the garden-variety tension type. They hurt, but they respond well to pain pills and lifestyle changes. Simply learning how to avoid or reduce the stress or other triggers is often all that is needed.

You May Have an Exertion Headache If . . .

- The pain begins when you're physically active: laughing, exercising, coughing, or having sex.

Exertion headaches may hit during or shortly after engaging in strenuous activity. They're not usually dangerous, but it's possible that they may be the sign of a stroke or other problem. It's best to get checked out just to make sure that these headaches are nothing more than an annoyance.

You May Have an Organic Headache If . . .

- The pain is new; that is, you haven't had this type of headache before.
- The pain is coupled with a fever, stiff neck, or other unusual symptoms.
- When the pain strikes, or soon after, there is confusion, difficulty moving or speaking, fatigue, or faintness.
- The pain begins after a head injury.
- The pain gets worse with each new headache, or headaches become more and more frequent.

Think of your headaches as you would a mole. That little mole on your arm probably isn't a serious problem unless it starts to change. That's when you must get it checked out by a physician. Just as you watch for changes in your moles, be aware of changes in your headache patterns. If you get the same headache every time you visit your in-laws, if it hurts as much and in the same way as it always does, it's probably just a tension headache. And if you suffer from the same head pain every time you eat MSG, you probably don't have to worry that you have a brain tumor. But, on the other hand, you shouldn't ignore these "stable" headaches. The odds are slim, but they just might be heralding a deeper problem. It's best to get yourself checked out by a physician, just to make sure.

There are many other types of headaches besides the tension, cluster, exertion, and organic types. You may, for example, be struck by headaches caused by low blood sugar, hangovers, constipation, or travel. Fortunately, solving the underlying problem can eliminate most of these headaches. But remember, it's always best to see your doctor if you're having any odd, unusually severe, or "different" headaches, just to be safe.

Migraine Miscellany

Money, school, and migraines. Well-educated and wealthy folk do not have any more migraines than those with less money or schooling. It only seems that way because those with more money and education tend to see doctors more often.

Migraines and stroke. A study in the May 2000 issue of *Neurology* reported that your risk of stroke might be higher if you have migraine headaches with aura. The migraines themselves are not the problem. Instead, it's the fact that some 50 percent of those who suffer from migraines also have an opening between the chambers of the heart called *foramen ovale.* Less than a third of the general population has this opening, which increases one's risk of suffering from an unusual type of stroke that strikes the young.

But don't worry: Even though people who have migraines *with* aura are three times more likely to suffer a stroke than those who have migraines *without* aura, and eight times more likely than the general population, the overall risk of stroke is still small for migraineurs.

The cost of migraines. Migraines cost a lot: People with migraines are responsible for twice as many medical and pharmaceutical insurance claims as nonsuffers.[1] And American taxpayers foot the bill for the approximately $13 billion in lost productivity due to migraines every year.[2]

Time lost to migraines. The typical migraineur loses between 1.4 and 4 days of work every year because of migraines.[3]

MIGRAINES ARE A REAL DISEASE
REQUIRING REAL HELP

Migraine is much more than a pain in the head: It's a constellation of symptoms affecting many parts of the body.

Migraines are not "all in your head." Despite the fact that they may sometimes seem to be related to stress, they are a genuine, physical problem.

Migraineurs require more than just a few aspirin, a ten-minute break, and a stern admonition to "buck up and get back to work!"

Migraines are not the only cause of severe head pain. Other types of headaches can hurt just as much.

It may take a while to get properly diagnosed. Sometimes doctors miss signs and symptoms. If you don't think your cur-

---

[1] "Impact of Migraines: Cost of Migraines." ACHENET (American Council for Headache Education). http://www.achenet.org/impact/cost.shtml.

[2] "Migraine Update." The National Institute of Neurological Disorders and Stroke. Reviewed August 21, 2000. http://www.ninds.nih.gov/health_and_medical/pubs/migraineupdate.htm.

[3] "Impact of Migraines: Cost of Migraines." ACHENET (American Council for Headache Education). http://www.achenet.org/impact/cost.shtml.

rent doctor is taking you seriously, you may have to find a new one.

It's worth the effort to get a diagnosis. True, up until now doctors haven't been able to help many migraine sufferers, and certainly haven't been able to "cure" the disease. But at last we have a new approach—the "triple therapy"—that may help make your headaches less frequent and less severe.

Chapter 3

———⟨O⟩———

New Hope from Nature

By the early 1990s, I had been treating people for their migraines and other headaches for over ten years, ever since my medical residency back in 1981. It was clear, however, that my doctor's little black bag didn't contain the medicine that millions of migraineurs were desperately seeking. In short, we doctors had nothing that could prevent future migraines, reliably, safely, and without side effects. I needed something new. And that something turned out to be the "triple therapy" I pioneered at my New York Headache Center.

This therapy consists of three very common natural substances: the mineral magnesium, the vitamin riboflavin (also known as vitamin B_2), and the herb feverfew. As a firm believer in establishing the science behind a treatment, I personally conducted a great deal of the published research that supports magnesium in the treatment of migraines. We'll delve into some of those studies, as well as the research on riboflavin and feverfew, in the next chapter. For now, let's step back to get an overview of the triple therapy, the new hope from nature that has helped many migraineurs.

THE BIRTH OF THE TRIPLE THERAPY

Ever since medical school, I have been interested in acupuncture, supplements, and other alternative methods. Even as I treated my patients with the approved medications of the day throughout the 1980s and into the 1990s, I kept my eye on various alternative approaches, reading articles as they appeared in the literature, asking questions of colleagues who were similarly intrigued, quizzing patients who told me they were trying supplements, acupuncture, or other modalities. (I have been performing acupuncture on patients since the 1980s.)

When it became clear that the standard medicines weren't able to provide the relief that my patients so desperately wanted, I began looking elsewhere in earnest. In 1992, I started studying the role of magnesium in migraine headaches with Burton Altura, Ph.D., professor of medicine at State University of New York and my laboratory-scientist colleague. The more research we conducted, the more I became convinced that this mineral could play an incredibly important role in migraine treatment and prevention.

Encouraged by the results of our migraine studies—plus my experience with patients—I decided to see if I could make the therapy even stronger by adding another ingredient. I knew that the herb feverfew was an effective treatment for many migraineurs, so I began giving it to some of my patients. I was also keeping an eye on riboflavin, which had been discussed as a potential treatment and preventive agent for migraines. But it wasn't until April 1997, when a double-blind study showing that riboflavin could indeed prevent migraines was published in the leading neurological journal *Neurology,* that I felt confident enough to begin working with it.

And so by 1997 the three elements of the triple therapy had come together, and the combination was soon helping many of my patients. Then, in December of that year, I was surprised to discover that a supplement containing magnesium, riboflavin, and feverfew had appeared on the market. Someone else had come up with the same combination and put it together in one pill. I started recommending this product to my patients. It worked, and it was easier to purchase the three supplements in one bottle rather than buy three different products—and it was much simpler to take two pills a day rather than the up to ten required with the three separate ingredients. Soon thereafter I was contacted by the researcher in Los Angeles who had formulated the product, and learned of the many migraineurs he had helped. Heartened to hear that the triple therapy was helping so many people, I forged ahead with more confidence, compiling more successful case histories as I gave these supplements to more and more patients.

It's been nine years since I began formulating my own triple therapy, and almost four since I completed my recipe. Given the number of scientific studies that support its use—and, more importantly, the tremendous number of people it's helped—I can confidently say that we've entered a new era of migraine treatment.

THREE COMMON INGREDIENTS
MAKE UP THE TRIPLE THERAPY

One of the nice things about using magnesium, riboflavin, and feverfew is that they're well-known, common substances that have been given to people for many years. Magnesium and riboflavin are found in many foods, play integral roles in general health, and are well tolerated by the human body. Indeed, the body stores a fair amount of magnesium in the bones. Feverfew, while not normally found in the human body, has been used by healers since at least the days of the ancient Greeks.

Caution: The ingredients in the triple therapy are common and generally well tolerated by humans, but anything—even water—can be dangerous in excess. Although we don't believe that humans can overdose on riboflavin, since the body eliminates any excess in the urine, we do know that taking excessive amounts of magnesium can upset the body's delicate biochemical balance. If you suffer from kidney disease or take an extraordinarily high dose of magnesium (measured in grams), you can suffer serious and potentially lethal side effects. Magnesium deficiency is more of a problem than magnesium excess, but it's best to be aware of the potential problems of overdose. Be sure to tell your physician that you are taking extra magnesium. As for feverfew, it can hamper blood clotting, which may be problematic for those who are taking anticoagulants or certain other medications. Also, if you chew on feverfew leaves, you may develop mouth ulcers. To be safe, it's best to consult with your physician before taking this or any other herb.

It is safe for children and pregnant women to take magnesium. However, we do not know what herbal remedies or high doses of riboflavin can do to developing fetuses or young children, so pregnant or nursing women, as well as young children, should be especially cautious about this or any other program, and work closely with their physicians.

Having said that, let's take a closer look at the ingredients in the triple therapy for migraine relief.

Ingredient #1: Magnesium

About 60 percent of the magnesium in the adult human body finds a home in the bones; the rest either resides in the cells or circulates through the bloodstream. Magnesium is a very popular participant in body chemistry, working with more than two hundred enzymes to help keep things running smoothly. This mineral helps the body:

- convert carbohydrates, protein, and fats into energy
- manufacture genetic material
- ensure that muscles contract and relax properly
- sweep away ammonia and other toxic substances
- transmit messages along the nerve pathways
- keep the teeth healthy
- keep the heart beating properly

It's very important that there be sufficient levels of magnesium in the blood at all times. Fortunately, if your blood levels fall below acceptable levels, the body is able to draw on the magnesium stored in the bones. Continually withdrawing from your "bone bank" isn't a good idea over the long run, but it will help you get through periods when you're not getting enough from your food, or your need for this mineral is greatly increased.

Magnesium functions as both the partner and opponent of calcium. Together, for example, they make it possible for muscles to function properly. Calcium helps them contract; magnesium lets them relax. The two minerals do the same for blood vessels. But magnesium and calcium must be kept in balance, or there will be trouble, for an excess of one of these minerals can trigger some of the same problems you'd see in a deficiency of the other. Suppose, for example, there's too much calcium relative to magnesium in the body. Without the relaxing effects of magnesium, blood vessels in the heart may contract too much, pinching off the flow of blood, possibly pushing blood pressure higher or kicking off a heart attack. On the other hand, taking in too much magnesium can make it difficult for your body to absorb enough calcium from your foods. But most magnesium-related problems are due to getting too little of this mineral rather than too much.

A lack of magnesium can lead to all kinds of problems, including:

- irregular heartbeats
- elevated blood pressure
- heart failure
- loss of appetite
- failure to grow
- insomnia
- muscle spasms
- "pins-and-needles" sensations in the hands and feet
- weakness
- shortness of breath
- convulsions
- nausea and other gastrointestinal problems
- poor coordination
- dizziness
- fatigue
- anxiety
- depression
- confusion
- premenstrual syndrome (PMS)

In severe cases, there may also be arterial damage, swelling of the gums, loss of hair, and perhaps even death.

Your body's store of magnesium might run low if you're not

getting enough in your diet. You may also run short if you have long-term diarrhea or vomiting, drink alcohol heavily, are using diuretic drugs for long periods of time, or have diabetes, kidney disease, or protein-calorie malnutrition. Then there's stress, a major depleter of magnesium. The detrimental effects of stress on the body's magnesium supply have been confirmed by many studies. In one involving a group of students, half were given a stressful test to take, while the other half were asked to read magazines. Then researchers measured the magnesium in the students' urine to see how much of the mineral was excreted. The results? The test-stressed students excreted much more magnesium than those who lounged about, reading.

We know that stress robs the body of magnesium. We also know stress can make migraines strike more frequently and more severely. When you put these two facts together, it appears that magnesium may be the biological link between stress and migraines—and possibly other conditions worsened by stress, as well.

Relatively few people are obviously and seriously deficient in magnesium, but smaller deficiencies are fairly common and uncommonly troublesome. Many Americans aren't meeting the RDA (recommended dietary allowance) for magnesium, which is 400 mg per day, and it's been estimated that 15–20 percent of Americans are chronically deficient.[1] And, in the case of migraine patients, there may be other problems. For example, if they're taking in too much calcium in their foods and/or supplements, they may not be able to absorb enough of the magnesium they consume. Or there may be problems with the way their bodies use magnesium. And physical and emotional stress may be causing them to "burn up" the magnesium they do take in.

[1]Durlach J, et al. "Magnesium and therapeutics." *Magnes Res* 7(3–4):313–28, 1994.

Where to Get Magnes[...]

Food	Serving size	
Whole wheat, cracked	1 cup	
Sunflower seeds	1 ounce	10[...]
Tofu	½ cup	94
Almonds	1 ounce	86
Hazelnuts	1 ounce	85
Cashew nuts	1 ounce	74
White beans, dry, cooked	½ cup	60
Broccoli, fresh, cooked	½ cup	47
Artichoke, cooked	1 medium	47
Skim milk	1 cup	36

Remember that while certain nuts are good sources of magnesium, they may also trigger migraines. If nuts are migraine triggers for you, look to other foods for your magnesium.

Ingredient #2: Riboflavin

A member of the B family of vitamins, riboflavin plays several roles in the body, assisting in:

- the release of energy from the carbohydrates, protein, and fats we eat
- normal growth

ber of hormones

...um
Milligrams of
magnesium

168

boflavin from
e vitamin from
ike magnesium,
ody, so you need
... Excess amounts of ri-
...n supplement form, are excreted
... bright yellow.
...rticipates in many bodily activities, so a defi-
... affect you in many different ways. A shortfall of this
...amin may cause:

- burning and soreness of the mouth, tongue and lips
- cracks in the corners of the mouth
- inflammation of the mucous membranes of the mouth
- poor vision
- light sensitivity
- red eyes
- dryness and other skin problems
- weakness
- fatigue
- conjunctivitis
- depression
- emotional difficulties
- mental difficulties

Small amounts of riboflavin are found in a variety of foods, so it's rare to see obvious and serious cases of deficiency. However, there are undoubtedly numerous people who take in barely adequate—or somewhat inadequate—amounts of this vitamin. The poor and elderly are especially likely to be deficient.[2] Fortunately, you don't have to worry about overdoing it, since whatever you don't need will simply be excreted. The RDA for riboflavin is 1.7 mg per day. However, it appears that some migraine sufferers need very large amounts of riboflavin because of a defect in the function of mitochondria, the energy generators for our cells.

Where to Get Riboflavin

Food	Serving size	Milligrams of riboflavin
Beef liver, braised	3 ounces	3.5
Calf liver, fried	3 ounces	3.5
Chicken liver, simmered	1 cup	2.4
Pork liver, braised	3 ounces	1.9
Milk, skim	1 cup	0.4
Wheat germ	½ cup	0.4
Yogurt, from skim milk	4 ounces	0.3
Mackerel, boneless, broiled	3 ounces	0.3
Egg	1 large	0.2
Bread, bran	1 slice	0.2

[2]Southon S, et al. "Micronutrient undernutrition in British schoolchildren." *Proc Nutr Soc* 52:155–63, 1993.

Ingredient #3: Feverfew

Over the past several years, many people have been surprised to learn that the herb with the odd-sounding name of feverfew can help relieve migraines and other headaches. This may seem like startling new information only because we've forgotten that as far back as 1649 a British herbalist noted that the herb was a good remedy for "all pains in the head." About 130 years after that, another British herbalist reported that feverfew was the best treatment for painful headaches, with a healing power that "exceeds whatever else is known." So feverfew is really a "brand-new old cure."

Unfortunately, feverfew, along with most other herbs, was swept aside by the tidal wave of drugs pouring out of pharmaceutical company laboratories in the middle part of the twentieth century. By the late 1950s it was all but forgotten. Then, in the late 1970s, reports of a woman who used feverfew to banish her migraine headaches appeared in British newspapers. In rapid succession, studies were published suggesting that the "new" herb did indeed lessen the pain of migraine headaches, and could perhaps prevent them from striking in the first place.

Besides headaches, feverfew is used today to treat arthritis, "female troubles," and many other ailments. You can purchase this herb in vitamin stores, health food stores, pharmacies, and supermarkets. (See chapter 5 for a few notes on purchasing feverfew.)

THE SCIENCE BEHIND THE TRIPLE THERAPY

As we entered the 1990s, we knew that magnesium and riboflavin were important nutrients, but that was of little interest to neurologists treating headaches. And the idea that feverfew might be helpful in treating migraines was not even mentioned in neurology journals. Few physicians treating migraines suspected that the mineral, the vitamin, and the herb would soon combine to offer an entirely new way of treating migraines and other headaches.

My medical school professors might be surprised to learn that I'm using these three natural substances to treat migraines. After all, I trained as a physician during the height of the pharmaceutical revolution; we gave barely a nod to vitamins and minerals, and never even glanced at herbs. Isn't it somehow unscientific to use these three substances instead of the latest drug? Can nutrients and herbs possibly be compared to "real" medicine?

Their use makes more sense if you recall that most of our early medicines were derived from nature, from herbs and foods. Scientific knowledge grew at a breathtaking pace in the twentieth century, so today our medicines are scientific-looking pills and capsules, intramuscular and intravenous injections. But there's still plenty of nature in our modern medications, many of which are highly refined versions of natural substances. Indeed, researchers from many of the high-tech pharmaceutical companies are scouring the tropical rain forests as you read this, looking for plants or herbs that have medicinal value and can be turned into modern drugs. So there's nothing unscientific about using a mineral, a vitamin, and an herb to relieve and prevent migraines. A medicine doesn't have to be a highly refined laboratory concoction to be considered good. It simply has to work, with a minimum of side effects. And that's exactly what the ingredients in my triple therapy do.

Let's take a look now at some of the science supporting the use of magnesium, riboflavin, and feverfew for migraines. This will just be an overview; we'll delve into the subject more thoroughly in the next chapter.

Magnesium and Migraines

About half the people who suffer from migraine headaches are deficient in a certain form of magnesium known as serum ionized magnesium, or "free" magnesium. There are two forms of magnesium in the body. One is inactive because it's bound to other substances. The other, the form we're concerned with, is *not* bound and *is* active. It's this free and active form that plays such an important role in causing or preventing migraines. When the free magnesium level drops:

- Blood vessels in the head are more likely to constrict, especially in the presence of substances like serotonin. This "clamping down" interrupts blood flow and may trigger a migraine.
- Various inflammatory substances in the brain are released, setting the stage for more pain and other symptoms.
- The blood vessels are less likely to relax on command from the body. This means that it's harder to get rid of the pain.

The magnesium/migraine link is very strong and quite well documented. We know, for example, that the same things that cause the body to run short of magnesium—menstruation, pregnancy, stress, alcohol, and certain diuretic drugs—can also trigger migraines. We also know that magnesium does many of the same helpful things that migraine medications do. For example, magnesium:

- Helps keep the blood vessels in the brain properly toned and open, allowing the blood to flow freely.
- Prevents the arteries from going into sudden spasm.
- Helps prevent platelets from sticking together inappropriately and causing "sludgy," slow-moving blood.

- Helps keep cell membranes stable.
- Interferes with substances in the body that cause inflammation.

In these ways, magnesium acts as a medicine for migraines.

It was first suggested that a deficiency of magnesium could cause headaches about seventy years ago, and up through the 1990s there were scattered reports of physicians using the mineral to relieve headaches. But only a few studies of magnesium were performed, yielding confusing results. That was because we could only measure total magnesium, not free magnesium.

When new techniques for measuring free magnesium were developed by Dr. Burton Altura in the early 1990s, my colleagues and I began studying the link between free magnesium and migraines. In 1993, I reported the results of a study with two hundred patients at my New York Headache Center.[3] We found that people suffering from acute migraines had lower levels of free magnesium in their blood. This finding was supported by another study in which we found that the level of free magnesium was low in 42 percent of those in the throes of a migraine attack.[4]

In 1995, my colleagues and I demonstrated that giving intravenous injections of magnesium to people with low levels of the mineral in their blood could relieve migraine headaches, often within 15 minutes.[5] And we found that the lower the

[3] Mauskop A, Altura B, Cracco R, Altura B. "Serum ionized magnesium levels in patients with tension-type headaches." In *Tension-type Headache: Classification, Mechanisms, and Treatment.* Olesen J and Schoenen J, eds. New York: Raven Press, 1993, 137–40.

[4] Mauskop A, Altura BT, Cracco RQ, Altura BM. "Deficiency in serum ionized magnesium but not total magnesium in patients with migraines. Possible role of $ICa^{2}+/IMg^{2}+$ratio." *Headache* 1993;33:135–38.

[5] Mauskop A, Altura B, Cracco R, Altura B. "Intravenous magnesium sulphate relieves migraine attacks in patients with low serum ionized magnesium levels: a pilot study." *Clinical Science* 1995; 89:633–36.

magnesium level when the migraine struck, the more dramatic and long-lasting the relief offered by the magnesium infusion.

In 1996, my colleagues and I studied the effects of magnesium in forty patients who came to the clinic with severe headaches of any type (not just migraine).[6] We found that giving 1 gram of magnesium intravenously completely eliminated the pain within 15 minutes in 80 percent of the volunteers—and associated symptoms, such as nausea and sensitivity to light, also vanished. In over half of the volunteers, the pain was still gone a day later. And those patients who enjoyed the best and longest-lasting response had the lowest levels of magnesium at the start. This study confirmed our previous findings: Low levels of magnesium are associated with migraines (and other headaches), and the lower the level of magnesium during the headache, the better the response to magnesium treatment.

My studies, those of other investigators, plus our success in treating hundreds of migraineurs made it clear that magnesium is a powerful new tool with which to fight migraines and other headaches.

What About Intravenous Magnesium Injections?

We know that taking magnesium orally, every day, can cut back on the number of migraines. Unfortunately, we also know that a small number of patients cannot tolerate oral magnesium: No matter which formulation is tried, it gives them diarrhea or stomach pain. For other people, supplements don't work because they can't absorb the mineral well or are not lacking in magnesium.

Doctors can measure their patients' magnesium levels to

[6] Mauskop A, Altura B, Cracco R, Altura B. "Intravenous magnesium sulfate rapidly alleviates headaches of various types." *Headache* 1996;36:154–60.

see if they're deficient, but the standard test is not very accurate, and the one we use in our studies is not readily available. Thus we sometimes use an intravenous injection of magnesium as a diagnostic tool, to see if patients are lacking in the mineral and if the shortfall is contributing to their migraines. If that is indeed the problem, the intravenous infusion usually offers dramatic and sudden relief—which may last for two to four weeks.

When faced with migraine patients who have not been helped by other means, most headache specialists will give an intravenous injection of magnesium. Our initial study at the New York Headache Center shows that this is an effective treatment for acute migraine attacks, a tremendous aid to the 50 percent of patients who have low magnesium levels.

I prefer to inject magnesium rather than other medications, for it has no serious side effects. I typically use 1 gram (sometimes 2) of magnesium sulfate diluted in saline. The magnesium opens up the blood vessels, which makes patients feel warm. It can also make them temporarily light-headed, so we make sure they're lying down. Potential side effects—which are very rare—include nausea and a strong sensation of flushing. Slowing the rate of infusion usually eliminates the problems.

Feverfew and Riboflavin for Migraines

Prized by ancient healers, then set aside and all but forgotten, feverfew was rediscovered in the latter part of the twentieth century. We don't know quite how it quells migraines: Our best hypothesis is that the parthenolide and other substances in the herb help dampen the inflammation process associated with migraines, as well as mitigate the effects of histamine and arachidonic acid that contribute to the headaches and their symptoms.

A 1985 study appearing in the British medical literature reported that when feverfew was withdrawn from people who were taking it to prevent migraines, their problems grew worse.[7] In 1988, British researchers published the results of a double-blind, placebo-controlled study involving some seventy migraineurs. (In a double-blind study, neither the researchers nor the participants know who is taking the feverfew and who is getting the placebo—the "sugar pill"—until the study is completed. This reduces the odds of the "placebo effect" coloring the results. See pages 60–61 for more on different types of studies.) The scientists found that taking feverfew led to a 24 percent drop in the frequency of attacks, and less nausea and vomiting. A 1999 report from Poland described what happened to twenty-four women given the herb for 30–60 days for their migraines: One-third enjoyed a significant reduction in migraine symptoms, and five others reported lesser improvements.[8] There were only slight side effects from feverfew.

Scientific studies are necessary and impressive, but there's nothing like real-life experience to confirm that a substance really helps. One of my favorite feverfew case histories, for which I can claim no credit, involves Debby. I met this forty-eight-year-old attorney at a dinner party. We were introduced by first name only; she didn't know I was a physician. A friend happened to ask how my book was going, Debby asked what the book was about, and I replied, "A new cure for migraines."

[7] Johnson ES, Kadam NP, Hylands, DM, Hylands, PJ. "Efficacy of feverfew as prophylactic treatment of migraine." *Br Med J (Clin Res Ed)* 1985 Aug 31;291 (6495):569–73.

[8] Prusinksi A, Durko A, Niczyporuk-Turek A. [Feverfew as a prophylactic treatment of migraine.] *Neurol Neurochir Pol* 1999;33 Suppl 5:89–95. [Article in Polish]

She instantly said, "I swear by feverfew! I can't go without it!"

"What kind of migraines do you get?" I asked.

"With aura. They're terrible. But I take feverfew every day, so I only get half as many as I used to and they only hurt half as much for half as long. I used to get migraines so terrible, they'd rush me to the emergency room to get one of those super-powerful drug shots. Now the feverfew takes care of it."

Thirty-five-year-old Don is one of the relatively small group of men with migraines. "I don't have an exciting story to tell," he said. "My headaches started when I was in college. They came once or twice a month for a year. They hurt a lot and I was nauseous, but luckily they didn't last very long. I didn't have any of those two- or three-day-long attacks. A friend from the dorms was into herbs. She told me about feverfew, so I tried it and I loved it. Since I started taking it thirteen years ago, I rarely get migraines."

Riboflavin, on the hand, has not been studied as intensely as feverfew or magnesium, but the reports that exist are quite encouraging. For example, a 1998 study of fifty-five migraineurs found that it was superior to placebo; it was better at reducing the number of migraine headaches. While there remains a great need for more research on riboflavin, it's clear that this common vitamin has an important role to play in the battle against migraines.

"I found out about riboflavin accidentally," explained forty-two-year-old Robin. "I had been having migraines for many years, and I was going from one medicine to another. Then I happened to go to a doctor for a complete checkup. Not for my migraines, but because my lips burned sometimes, and had cracks in the corners, and my tongue was sore sometimes. He didn't find any disease, but thought my problem might be due to a lack of B vitamins. He suggested I change my diet and take lots of B vitamins. I did, and several months later noticed I wasn't getting as many migraines. We experimented a bit, and figured out that the riboflavin in the B vitamins was taking care of my migraines and my mouth problems."

THE PROOF IS IN THE PATIENTS

Taken separately, magnesium, riboflavin, and feverfew have strong effects. When you put them all together, you're "covering all the bases" by correcting multiple problems that can lead to migraines. Here are some of my "triple therapy" successes:

Blanche is a seventy-five-year-old woman who has been suffering from migraines for some sixty years. She began taking the triple therapy one year ago and found it to be very effective. "I used to have several migraines a week, but haven't had one for six months. Sometimes I get the aura, but the headache just doesn't develop. And even the auras are getting fewer and further in between."

Sixty-five-year-old Shirley has also been suffering from migraines since she was a teenager. "I used to cry to my mother when I got them." Unfortunately, Shirley has heart disease, which means she can't use Imitrex or certain other migraine medications. "I was having a migraine every other day. I thought I was going to go out of my mind. Then I heard about magnesium, riboflavin, and feverfew. After I took the therapy for about one month, my headaches started getting less frequent. Now I only get one every other week, and it's not as severe as it used to be."

Kristen is a twenty-eight-year-old woman who has suffered from migraines for about eight years now. "I would get a migraine about two or three times a week. Since I never knew when the next one would hit, my life was constantly interrupted. I was forever canceling plans because of those migraines. I tried many medicines, but either they didn't help or the side effects from the pills were severe, so I never stayed on one drug for very long. Meanwhile, the doctor bills were piling up. Tired of getting no relief, I decided to look for a more natural approach. I came across that combination of magnesium, feverfew, and riboflavin called MigraHealth™ (also sold as MigraLief®). About a month later, I couldn't believe it— my migraines were coming less often. Over the next couple of months, they disappeared almost entirely. I've been taking the triple therapy for two years now, and it's really been great."

MIGRAINES . . . AND MORE?

Migraineurs may not be the only headache patients who can benefit from magnesium. Some of the volunteers in early studies of the mineral had suffered from cluster headaches—and some of them, like many of the migraineurs, had low levels of magnesium. This led us to wonder: Could cluster headaches also be related to lack of magnesium? These headaches occur in clusters or groups, sometimes daily for a period of up to two to three months every year, with each attack lasting one to two hours. Unlike migraines, cluster headaches prefer to strike men.

Would supplemental magnesium help relieve their problems? If so, it would be a tremendous boon to the many who suffer from what have been dubbed "suicide headaches," because the pain is so terrible that some patients consider—and a few even attempt—ending their lives.

In 1994, my colleagues and I conducted a study on sixteen patients suffering from either episodic or chronic cluster headaches.[9] We found that half of those suffering from episodic cluster headaches had low levels of free magnesium and had relatively high amounts of free calcium compared to free magnesium. This was a small study, but it suggested that magnesium might play a role in certain people who suffer from cluster headaches, and that supplementation might help alleviate the problem. We followed this up with another study on twenty-two cluster headache patients, who were given intravenous infusions of magnesium.[10] Nine of the volunteers (41 percent) reported improvement that lasted for at least two days—and the elimination of at least two expected cluster attacks.

We need to conduct more, larger, and more scientifically rigorous studies to test the magnesium/cluster theory, and to rule out the placebo effect or spontaneous remission. Still, these preliminary studies are intriguing, and may point to a new, successful, and safe method of relieving and/or preventing cluster headaches in certain people.

I remember well one of my cluster patients, a stockbroker named Steven, whose cluster headaches were stopped in their tracks by an infusion of magnesium and didn't return for two weeks.

Even more dramatic is the story of John, who stumbled into my office with a "killer cluster," demanding instant relief. I gave him an infusion of magnesium rather than an injection of a pain-killing drug. Almost immediately, his headache went away, and it didn't come back until the next year's cycle of clusters began. While one may think his cluster cycle ended naturally,

[9] Mauskop A, Altura BT, Cracco RQ, Altura BM. "Ionized Mg, total Mg, and ICa^{2+} ratios in patients with episodic (ECH) and chronic (CCH) cluster headaches." *Headache Quarterly, Current Treatment and Research* 1994;5(2):156–58.

[10] Mauskop A, Altura BT, Cracco RQ, Altura BM. "Intravenous magnesium sulfate relieves cluster headaches in patients with low serum ionized magnesium levels." *Headache* 1995;35:597–600.

his cycles typically lasted six to eight weeks. The magnesium ended his headaches when he was only one week into the cycle!

NATURAL, SAFE, AND EFFECTIVE

After almost nine years of scientific study building on earlier theory and research programs, plus experience with hundreds of patients, I can confidently say that the triple therapy is a new approach to preventing migraine and possibly other headaches. The therapy has stood the most important test of all—the patient test. Many patients had not been helped by the strongest drugs and best therapies available. If the triple therapy can help them, it just might help you, too. Perhaps the best part is that the triple therapy is very natural and safe, and it's just a part of my larger program for treating and preventing these terrible headaches.

If you'd like to learn more about the science behind the triple therapy, keep reading. If you'd prefer to jump right into the Banishing Migraines Program, skip to chapter 5.

Chapter 4

───────◄○►───────

Inside the Triple Therapy

Many a doctor dealing with headaches up through the early 1990s must have felt as I did: like a handyman trying to fix a rickety old house. Unfortunately, I wasn't allowed to go into the house to examine the woodwork, pipes, and wires personally; I couldn't take measurements or samples. Instead, I was only permitted to investigate from the outside. Standing several feet back from the house, I could see that the wood and bricks were old and worn. I could walk around the outside, knock on the water pipes that went in and out of the structure, touch the siding and check the exterior paint, notice broken windows, and take copious notes. But since I wasn't allowed to go inside, I couldn't check the foundation or get at the hidden plumbing and electrical wiring. Neither could I take samples of the interior wood to check for termites or rot. The best I could do was make some educated guesses, then tell the workmen to pour a bunch of cement over here or nail on some new siding over there. Sometimes it worked, but lots of times it didn't.

Until recently, we doctors weren't able to help our migraineurs and other headache patients nearly as well as we—and certainly they—would have liked. We had several thorny problems, including these:

- Our primary method of classifying headaches, the International Headache Society (IHS) classification, missed a lot of people. It was unable to account for a significant proportion of patients who didn't fit neatly into certain predetermined categories.
- Even when it did "capture" the patients, the IHS classification was only descriptive. That is, it might tell us that someone was suffering from a migraine or cluster headache, but could not predict which treatment would work best—or work at all.
- Our primary tools, our drugs, didn't help everyone. They couldn't even help *most* people. Even when you added in our other tools, such as bed rest, cold compresses, and biofeedback, we weren't terribly successful. Only a minority of patients—some one-third—were fully satisfied with the treatments we offered. The other two-thirds were unhappy.
- We weren't getting to all the people. As many as 60 percent of migraineurs were undiagnosed and without medical treatment.
- In one sense it was a good thing that so many people went untreated, since the medications we can prescribe can be harmful to many people. The side effects of our standard migraine drugs include nausea, rapid heart rate, elevated blood pressure, weakness, dizziness, vertigo, numbness, itching, flushing, pain and stiffness in the neck, and sore throat.

Doctors had strong theories about migraines; we were pretty sure that they were related to the inappropriate "squeeze and release" of blood vessels and neurochemical changes in the brain. We felt that serotonin and nitric oxide played important roles in the genesis of a migraine, and that stress and numerous other triggers could turn a peaceful head into what felt like "a punching bag after Mike Tyson is finished practicing" or "a hockey puck in the midst of the Stanley Cup finals."

By the early 1990s we had taken several steps forward in the treatment of migraines, with powerful new drugs capable of stopping even severe attacks, but we were stuck when it came to migraine prevention. We hadn't solved the problem, and we weren't sure where to go next. What new theory would arise? What new treatment?

The new idea turned out to be an old one: the combination of magnesium, riboflavin, and the herb feverfew.

A Few "Study" Terms

It helps to know a few of the terms researchers toss around when discussing studies.

Placebo-controlled means that some of the people in a study are getting the real medicine, the others a placebo. A placebo is a "sugar pill," a substance with no medicinal value that's used as a basis of comparison. If the medicine being studied isn't significantly more effective than a placebo, it's probably not worth taking. Interestingly enough, a sizable portion of people taking placebos improve, apparently because they believe they're getting the real thing. Their thoughts act like a medicine. This is called the placebo effect.

If a study if *blind*, that means that someone doesn't know something. In a *single-blind* study, the patients don't know if they're getting the medicine or the placebo until the end of the study. In a *double-blind* study, neither the doctors nor the patients know who is getting what until it's all over.

If no one knows who is taking the real medicine, how does a double-blind study work? A third party assigns code numbers or letters to the participants and determines who gets what. This third party decides, for example, that patients 1, 3, 4, 6, and 8 get magnesium, while patients 2, 5, 7, 9, and 10 get the placebo. When the study is completed, the third party "breaks the code" and the researchers can match up the results with the participants.

In a *crossover study*, the patients receive one treatment for a certain amount of time, then another for an additional term. For example, they may get magnesium injections weekly for 10 weeks, followed by 10 weeks of injections with a similar-looking saltwater solution (a placebo).

An *open study* has no placebo-taking group, is not blinded, and has no crossover. The participants simply take the substances being studied. Everyone knows what he or she is taking, which means that the placebo effect may skew the results.

A placebo-controlled study is considered more scientifically valid than an open study, for it gives the researchers a standardized, known factor (the placebo) against which to compare the results. A double-blind study is considered more valid than a single-blind or open study, for it reduces the chances of subjective feelings on the part of the patients or doctors changing the outcome. Even better is a double-blind, placebo-controlled crossover study.

MAGNESIUM FOR MIGRAINES

The idea that magnesium might play a role in migraines and other headaches is not new; in fact, it was first suggested way back in the early 1930s. In 1933, the prestigious British medical journal *Lancet* published a report of the successful use of magnesium injections to prevent one patient's migraine headaches.[1] Since then, there have been many reports of people who have been helped by magnesium. But the middle of the twentieth century saw the flowering of the pharmaceutical industry. As drugs began to conquer one disease after another, many doctors scoffed at the idea that a simple nutrient had medicinal value. Magnesium and other natural remedies were swept aside and largely forgotten.

Long dormant, the idea that a lack of magnesium might cause migraines—and that supplemental magnesium might help—was revived in the middle and late 1980s. In 1990, the journal *Headache* published the results of a study involving more than three thousand volunteers suffering from migraine with or without aura.[2] The patients, most of whom were women of childbearing age, were given about 200 mg of magnesium daily. The researchers reported an 80 percent success rate. Unfortunately, it wasn't clear what constituted success, and this was an open trial, not the double-blind, placebo-controlled study that's considered more scientifically valid.

This study was followed a year later by another report in *Headache* of a double-blind study of twenty-four women suffering from menstrual migraines.[3] Some of these women were given 360 mg of magnesium per day, from the fifteenth day of

---

[1] Pines N, et al. "Magnesium sulphate in the treatment of angiospasm." *Lancet* 1933;1:577–79.

[2] Weaver K. "Magnesium and migraine." *Headache* 1990;30:168.

[3] Facchinetti F, et al. "Magnesium prophylaxis of menstrual migraine: effects on intracellular magnesium." *Headache* 1991;31:298–301.

their cycles until menstruation, for two months. The other women in the study received placebos according to the same schedule. The women in the magnesium group enjoyed a significant reduction in the "Pain Total Index" (a measure of the length and intensity of their headaches), and had fewer headache days, compared to those getting the placebo.

By the early 1990s, it seemed clear that magnesium was linked to many migraines and other headaches. But we were like puzzle-solvers just starting out. A huge pile of puzzle pieces was dumped on the table upside down and right side up. They were lying helter-skelter on top of each other and we could only fit a few of them together. For example, we knew that:

- The total magnesium level was low in the midst of a migraine but not a tension-type headache.
- There was less magnesium in the serum, red blood cells, or certain white blood cells of migraine patients—according to some studies, but not others.
- Magnesium levels were lower in the brain during and between migraine attacks—in some people.
- Giving magnesium to headache patients was very helpful—in many patients.

Those caveats—"according to some studies," "in some people," and "in many patients"—kept popping up. Why? This should be a simple equation: Either low magnesium equals migraines, and supplemental magnesium solves the problem, or it doesn't. But things weren't factoring out quite so simply.

As better laboratory tests became available, we learned why the magnesium/migraine equation didn't work out the same way in every study. We were being confused by the fact that all magnesium in the body is *not* the same. Whether in the cells or in blood fluid, the mineral comes in different forms: It may be bound to other substances and inactive, or unbound and active ("free"). Up until recently, we've only been able to measure the total magnesium (TMg), which is made up of the types of magnesium combined. That's where the confusion arose, since the total magnesium turned out to be less important than the amount of serum ionized magnesium (IMg^{2+}), or free magnesium.

A Few Definitions

Serum is the clear fluid in the blood in which the cells float, proteins are dissolved, etc. If you let blood clot, what's left is a yellowish fluid called *blood serum.*

An *ion* is an atom or group of atoms that have gained or lost electrons, leaving them with positive or negative electrical charges.

Size, Form, and Charge Affect Function

Isn't magnesium always magnesium, even if it's temporarily hooked on to something else? Or if it's bent out of shape a little, or has one too many or one too few electrons? Not according to the body. Size, shape, and electrical charge are very important on a biochemical level. Everything has to be in just the right form, because body chemistry works on a "lock-and-key" system.

We believed that magnesium could help blood vessels in the brain relax, among other things. But we knew that in order for that to happen, the magnesium "key" had to fit perfectly into the "lock" that, when turned, released tension in the vessels. If there was just one little flaw or difference in the magnesium key, it wouldn't fit into the lock.

This means that size is vital. Something as simple as being bound to another atom or molecule can make the magnesium key too big, and thus inoperative. Suppose there's a small window in your house, just big enough to allow your ten-year-old son to wriggle through. He comes home from school one day and discovers that he's forgotten his house key. No problem. He opens the little window and squeezes through. Your son is a perfect fit, size-wise, for the window. He's the "key"; the window is the "lock." Now imagine that he comes home from school one day, again without his key—but this time he has a backpack full of books on his back. He again opens the window and tries to squeeze through, but he can't. With the backpack strapped on, he's too big. He has to take the pack off, wriggle through the opening, then reach through the window to pull the backpack in along with him. In our world, it's easy to add or subtract backpacks and other things that make us temporarily too large to fit through openings. But in the biochemical world it's not so simple. Magnesium that is bound to something else is like your son with a backpack: It doesn't fit through the opening anymore. Unable to get through that opening to do its biochemical job, it can't perform properly.

Shape is just as important as size in the tiny world of body chemistry. We rarely think about the shape of an atom or molecule. After all, when you look at a diagram of an atom or molecule in a chemistry book, it's two-dimensional and flat. The C's representing carbon atoms are connected by lines to the O's signifying oxygen atoms, the H's designating hydrogens, and so on. From the picture, you would have no idea that the substance has a three-dimensional shape. But atoms and molecules have very definite, very specific three-dimensional shapes. A little change anywhere in the makeup can change the shape. Suppose you want to buy a can of soda from a machine. You fish some coins out of your purse or pocket and drop them into the machine one by one. Whoops! The last coin is very slightly bent, so the machine refuses to accept it. The coin "key" that should unlock the soda machine "lock" doesn't work, and you can't get your soda, all because of a tiny change in the coin's three-dimensional shape.

And finally, electrical charge is also very important. Electrons, as you remember from chemistry class, are negatively charged particles "in orbit" around atoms such as magnesium. Although atoms have a standard allotment of electrons, they can often take on an additional one, or let one go. When that happens, the electrical charge changes. Is that really important? Well, what happens when you put the negative end of a magnet next to the positive end of another magnet? They attract each other. And what happens when you place two positive or two negative ends together? They repel, they push away from each other. Something similar happens in the body; that's why the electrical charge is so important. An ionized atom, one that has taken on or dropped off an electron, has a different charge and attracts, or works with, other substances differently. The wrong charge can make a substance useless for one task, but absolutely perfect for another. Change the charge and you change the suitability.

New Techniques Provide Clues

By 1992, new laboratory techniques developed by Drs. Burton Altura and Bella Altura allowed us to measure more than the total magnesium (TMg) in the blood. We could now look at the serum ionized magnesium (IMg^{2+}), a form of free magnesium configured differently than the "standard" variety. Now, at last, we could measure the parts that went into the making of the total magnesium count. It was as if, up until then, we could only say, "You've got ten dollars worth of coins in your piggy bank." Now we could go beyond that to report, "You have three hundred pennies, twenty nickels, thirty dimes, and twelve quarters, for a total of ten dollars in your piggy bank."

Does it really matter that we can break down the coins that way? They still add up to ten dollars, so what's the difference? Think about how specific coins can be. You can't put ten pennies into a parking meter; you have to use two nickels or one dime. And seventy-five pennies won't do you any good if the candy machine requires nickels, dimes, or quarters. If you are trying to buy candy out of a machine, having a "total coin value" of ten dollars is worthless if the coins are all silver dollars or pennies. As far as the machine is concerned, the silver dollars and pennies are "inert," while the other coins are "active." You need to know what goes into the making of that total—how many pennies, quarters, etc.—before you can tell if you're going to get your candy.

Thanks to the new laboratory techniques, we could also look at the ratio between serum ionized magnesium and serum ionized calcium (ICa^{2+}). The balance between this form of magnesium and this form of calcium is important, for minerals and other substances interact in the body. Often, they're "opposed" by another mineral or substance. For example, calcium helps build strong bones, but taking in too much magnesium can interfere with the formation of bones. And while calcium stimulates muscles, encouraging them to contract, magnesium does the opposite, helping them relax. We need a certain balance between calcium and magnesium, so that muscles can squeeze when necessary, then release. Too much calcium compared to magnesium, for example, may lead to excessive muscle squeezing. Having a little less of one substance is like having too much of the other. For this reason, the calcium/magnesium ratio is as important as the absolute amount of either mineral. Here's another way to think of it: If you have either too much pasta or too much marinara sauce, your spaghetti is no good. You have to have the right balance, the right ratio of pasta to sauce, if you want a tasty meal.

Serum Ionized Magnesium Is the Key Migraine Culprit

Armed with the new laboratory techniques, my colleagues and I set out to learn whether a lack of serum ionized magnesium might be the real migraine culprit, and what role was played by the ratio of serum ionized magnesium to serum ionized calcium.

For this study, we used more than a hundred consecutive patients at my New York Headache Center.[4] The volunteers were divided into two groups: those with intermittent migraines, and those with continuous headaches. We also had sixty people who did not suffer from migraines serving as a control group, to be used for comparison. We began by drawing blood samples from the patients and healthy controls, then sending the samples to the laboratory for analysis. We deliberately didn't send any information about the study participants along with the samples; nobody was to know who had what levels of which substances until the end of the study.

When we looked at the results of the blood tests, and matched them up with the study volunteers, we found:

[4] Mauskop A, Altura BT, Cracco RQ, Altura BM. "Deficiency in serum ionized magnesium but not total magnesium in patients with migraines. Possible role of ICa^{2+}/IMg^{2+} ratio." *Headache* 1993;33:135–38.

- Forty-two percent of those with migraines had low serum ionized magnesium, plus an elevated ratio of serum ionized calcium to serum ionized magnesium. In other words, they had less of the specific, key kind of magnesium, and too much calcium compared to that magnesium.
- Only 23 percent of those with the severe continuous headaches had similar levels of serum ionized magnesium and serum ionized calcium.
- Both groups, however, had normal levels of total magnesium in their blood serum. (This is one of the things that had been confusing us before we were also able to measure the serum ionized magnesium.)
- Even among those with normal total magnesium, however, it was on the low end of normal in those who also had low serum ionized magnesium. The total magnesium levels weren't low enough to raise suspicions, but when combined with the low serum ionized magnesium, a pattern emerged.

These results helped clarify the picture. Magnesium *was* a factor in headaches. But the key was serum ionized magnesium, not total magnesium. Total magnesium, in fact, might be within normal limits, albeit on the low side. This study helped explain the confusing results of previous studies, and pointed us in a new, more narrowly focused direction.[5]

Intravenous Magnesium Relieves Migraines

By 1995, we knew from my experiments and the work of other investigators that a lack of serum ionized magnesium seemed to trigger migraines in many people. We were eager to

---

[5] See the Appendix for information on the follow-up study we conducted to confirm these results.

push the magnesium-migraine connection one step further by showing that giving the mineral to patients who were lacking in it could help treat migraines.

Many case histories and one double-blind, placebo-controlled study had already suggested that oral doses of magnesium helped relieve migraines—in some people. We wanted to discover exactly which people would be helped the most, and we suspected it was those with lower levels of serum ionized magnesium.

To prove that this was so, we performed a study on 40 consecutive patients who were having migraines at the time of their visits to our center.[6] Of the thirty-seven women and three men, seven had migraines with aura, and thirty-three had migraines without aura. They ranged in age from twenty-three to fifty-eight.

After informing them of what we planned to do, we drew blood samples to check for total magnesium, serum ionized magnesium, and serum ionized calcium. Next, we asked them to rate their headaches on a scale of 1 to 10, with 10 being the absolute worst. Finally, the patients were given infusions of 1 gram of magnesium sulphate ($MgSO_4$ in a 10 percent solution given over 5 minutes).

It's important to emphasize that this was a blind study. We drew their blood to check for magnesium and other items, but did not know the results of the blood tests before we gave them the IV magnesium. All forty volunteers were given the magnesium infusions, even those who later turned out to have adequate levels of magnesium. We even made sure that the laboratory technicians measuring the blood knew nothing

[6] Mauskop A, Altura AT, Cracco RQ, Altura BM. "Intravenous magnesium sulphate relieves migraine attacks in patients with low serum ionized magnesium levels: a pilot study." *Clinical Science* 1995;89:633–36.

about the subjects—they didn't even know the names of the volunteers. This was done to help ensure that personal opinions about the mineral wouldn't influence the study one way or the other.

After giving the patients the magnesium, we asked them to rate their pain on a 1–10 scale twice more: 15 minutes after they got the IV magnesium, and again, by telephone, 24 hours later.

As we expected, the magnesium stopped a lot of migraine pain right away. In thirty-five of the forty patients (87.5 percent), pain levels dropped by half or more within 15 minutes. And nine reported that their migraine pain disappeared completely! Of the thirty-five who responded positively to the magnesium infusion, twenty-one were still headache-free 24 hours later.

We had expected the intravenous magnesium to relieve migraine pain. But did those people who had low levels of serum ionized magnesium to begin with benefit more than the others, as we had hoped?

To see if that was indeed true, 24 hours after the infusion we separated the twenty-one patients who were still feeling better from the nineteen who were not. Then we looked at the blood we drew at the beginning of the study to see who had low serum ionized magnesium to begin with and who did not.

Eighteen of the twenty-one who still felt better 24 hours later began with low magnesium.[7] But only three of the nineteen who did *not* feel better 24 hours later began with low magnesium. Our initial hypothesis was correct! This showed that there was indeed a very strong relationship between headache reduction and low serum ionized magnesium. Those who had low serum ionized magnesium to begin with were much more

---

[7] This was defined as an IMg^{2+} below 0.54 mmol/L.

likely to respond positively to the magnesium infusion than those with high serum ionized magnesium.

Why is this so significant? Because it goes beyond proving that magnesium helps relieve migraines. It tells us that the people with low magnesium are the ones most likely to benefit from extra magnesium. This is very important, because nothing helps everyone. That's why, for example, doctors may first try one painkiller then another on a given patient, before finding the most effective drug. But if you know ahead of time who is most likely to benefit, you can save people a lot of time—and a lot of pain—by selecting the best medicine right away.

The side effects from the IV magnesium were very minor: A flushed feeling while getting the infusion was reported by all forty patients, and twelve were light-headed for a few minutes when they sat up after the IV. Remember, however, that this was from magnesium injected right into the veins, not from magnesium tablets.

Another Magnesium Migraine Study

My colleagues and I performed a similar study the following year, using twenty-nine women and eleven men, ranging in age from fourteen to fifty-five.[8] Of the forty volunteers, sixteen had migraines without aura, fifteen had chronic migrainous headaches, and nine suffered from cluster headaches. As in the previous study, we explained the procedure to the volunteers, drew blood to test for ionized magnesium and other tests, asked them to rate their headaches on a scale of 1 to 10, and gave them an intravenous infusion of magnesium sulfate.

In thirty-two of the forty patients, the pain rating initially

[8] Mauskop A, Altura BT, Cracco RQ, Altura BM. "Intravenous magnesium sulfate rapidly alleviates headaches of various types." *Headache* 1996;36:154–60.

dropped by at least 50 percent. And in 80 percent of these thirty-two patients, the pain was completely gone 15 minutes after they received the IV magnesium. Not only was the pain gone, the nausea and light sensitivity that so often accompany migraines had also vanished. Eighteen of the thirty-two who initially responded to the magnesium were still enjoying headache relief 24 hours later.

Now it was time to "break the code," to look at the results of the blood tests we took at the beginning of the study. Which of the volunteers had low magnesium levels? Were the ones with low magnesium most likely to respond to the extra magnesium we pumped into their bodies?

Fortunately, the answer was yes. Of the eighteen people who were still feeling fine 24 hours later, fourteen began with a serum ionized level of 0.54 mmol/L or lower. (Normal levels are above 0.54.) In other words, if their magnesium was low to begin with, they were likely to benefit—quite a bit—from the magnesium infusion. When we published the results of our study in the journal *Headache,* we noted that "Overall, in 75 percent of the patients there was a correlation between the clinical response to intravenous $MgSO_4$ and the serum IMg^{2+} level." Our results were confirmed by a Turkish study published in 2001. This single-blind study showed that 87 percent of fifteen patients receiving 1 gram of intravenous magnesium obtained complete pain relief, while none of the fifteen patients in the placebo group obtained such relief.[9]

[9] Demirkaya S, Vural O, Dora B, et al. "Efficacy of intravenous magnesium sulfate in the treatment of acute migraine attacks." *Headache* 2001;41:171–77.

You Don't Have to Get an IV—Magnesium Supplements Also Work

It was clear that intravenous infusions of magnesium could stop migraines and other types of headaches in their tracks. But rushing to the doctor's office every time your head begins to throb is inconvenient—not to mention expensive. Is there a simpler way? Can magnesium supplements do just as well as intravenous injections? An Italian study on twenty-four women suffering from menstrual migraines suggested that they can, but this study was fairly small.

Researchers in Germany put the question to the test in a larger, 16-week study of eighty-one migraine patients, ranging in age from eighteen to sixty-five.[10] The volunteers had either migraines with aura or migraines without aura, and suffered through a mean of 3.6 migraines per month. The study was double-blind, randomized, and placebo-controlled.

The first 4 weeks were the baseline period: The patients were given neither magnesium nor the placebo; they were simply monitored. For the next 12 weeks, those in the magnesium group took a powdered preparation containing 600 mg of magnesium,[11] while those in the placebo group took a powder that did not contain the mineral. Throughout the study period, the volunteers kept diaries recording the number of migraines they experienced, their length and intensity, any medication they took, and side effects they suffered. The side effects of the magnesium, noted by a few patients, were gastric distress and diarrhea.

The results were impressive. The number of attacks, the

[10] Peikert A, Wilimzig C, Kohne-Volland R. "Prophylaxis of migraine with oral magnesium: results from a prospective, multi-center, placebo-controlled and double-blind randomized study." *Cephalalgia* 1996;16:257–63.

[11] Trimagnesium dicitrate, Magnesium Diasporal N 300.

number of days lost to migraines, and the amount of drugs necessary to treat the problem dropped significantly in the magnesium group. In the researcher's own words, "We have demonstrated that a high oral dose of magnesium lowered the frequency of migraine attacks within 12 weeks of therapy." In other words, here was proof that magnesium, taken orally, could help migraine patients by preventing the attacks from striking in the first place.

Another double-blind study, performed in Europe and described in the journal *Cephalalgia* in 1996, came up with negative results.[12] However, this study had a major flaw. The magnesium formulation chosen was poorly absorbed and caused diarrhea: 45 percent of patients who received magnesium developed diarrhea, while only 22 percent on placebo suffered similarly. (Certain magnesium salts are not well absorbed and, in fact, are used as laxatives.) This study is important in that it points out the importance of using a type of magnesium the body can tolerate well.

Magnesium and Menstrual Migraines

I've already mentioned the 1991 Italian study on twenty-four women suffering from menstrual migraines.[13] Doses of only 360 mg of magnesium reduced the number of headache days, the length and the intensity of the attacks.

My colleagues and I conducted our own small study of menstrual migraines at my New York Headache Center in

[12] Pfaffenrath V, Wessely P, Meyer C, et al. "Magnesium in the prophylaxis of migraine—A double-blind, placebo-controlled study." *Cephalalgia* 1996; 16:436–440.

[13] Facchinetti F, et al. "Magnesium prophylaxis of menstrual migraine: effects on intracellular magnesium." *Headache* 1991;31:298–301.

1997.[14] We worked with two volunteers whose serum ionized magnesium remained low, despite the fact that they were taking oral supplements. Every month, about a week before the onset of menstruation, they were each given intravenous infusions of 1 or 2 grams of magnesium ($MgSO_4$). The results were gratifying: The magnesium both prevented the menstrual migraines *and* relieved PMS symptoms. Over the years, I have given intravenous infusions to many women who suffer from menstrual migraines. Not only were their menstrual migraines prevented or significantly ameliorated, but in many cases their PMS symptoms were eliminated as well. (The researchers in the 1991 Italian study also noted that magnesium relieved PMS symptoms.)

The Theory behind the Practice

It's clear that low levels of magnesium are linked to migraine headaches in a great many people. But not just any magnesium: specifically serum ionized magnesium. The ratio between serum ionized magnesium and serum ionized calcium is also an important factor.

And now for the million-dollar question: Why? As is so often true in medicine, the answer is that we're not quite sure. This much we do know: Several items that trigger migraines, such as alcohol and stress, also cause the body to lose magnesium. Could these trigger items be setting off the migraines indirectly, by lowering the body's store of the mineral?

We also know that magnesium affects the body like certain drugs we have used to treat or prevent migraines. Specifically, magnesium:

---

[14] Mauskop A, Altura BT, Cracco RQ, Altura BM. "Intravenous magnesium for the prophylaxis of menstrual migraines." *Cephalalgia* 1997;17:425.

- helps blood vessels that have "squeezed" to "release" themselves
- slows the aggregation of platelets
- stabilizes cell membranes
- slows the body's inflammation process
- alters the function of serotonin and other brain receptors

Given that magnesium can behave like a medicine, and that it helps to slow the cascade of body reactions that take place at the birth of a migraine, it's fair to hypothesize that a lack of magnesium is at the root of the problem.

Don't let the open questions about magnesium alarm you, though. In truth, we're not sure how a lot of things in the body work. Neither can we completely explain why many of our standard medications are effective, including drugs we've used for years and years. We simply know that they do, and there's no arguing with success.

A Brief Word on Children

Watching a child suffer from migraines can be heartbreaking. The invisible pain that grips his or her head grips your heart as well. And there's always a special concern when dealing with youngsters, for the medicines we give to adults are sometimes inappropriate or even dangerous for children. Fortunately, magnesium can be just as helpful to children as it is to adults. In a study of eighty-six children suffering from frequent migraines, magnesium was pitted against a placebo.[15] The magnesium produced a statistically significant reduction in the number and

---

[15] Wang F, Van Den Eden S, Ackerson L, Salk S, Reince R. "Oral magnesium oxide prophylaxis of frequent childhood migraine." *Cephalalgia* 2000;20:424.

severity of migraines among the children, who ranged in age from three to seventeen.

FEVERFEW FOR MIGRAINES

The second member of my triple therapy is feverfew. Known scientifically as *Tanacetum parthenium,* this herb has been used to treat inflammation, fever, and "women's problems" for many years. More recently, this relative of the daisy has been put to work preventing migraine headaches.

The herb's name comes from the Latin for "chases away fevers," and a look at surviving Greek writings shows that it was also used for swelling, inflammation, and menstrual problems. Later British herbalists used the herb to quell headaches and fevers and to relieve the pain of arthritis, but feverfew and many other herbs were all but discarded during the rise of modern drug-based medicine. Only recently, in the last few decades of the twentieth century, did interest in the herb revive. Today, it's approved in both Canada and Britain for use in treating migraines, and the herb is being studied in various countries. For example, during the mid-1990s, researchers at the Center for Migraine Therapy in Poland studied twenty-four women, ranging in age from nineteen to sixty-one.[16] The volunteers were given feverfew once a day for 30–60 days, and their migraine symptoms were catalogued. The researchers found that the migraine symptoms were significantly reduced in eight of the twenty-four, while another five enjoyed smaller improvements.

---

[16] Prusinski A, Durko A, Niczyporuk-Turek A. [Feverfew as a prophylactic treatment of migraine]. *Neurol Neurochir Pol* 1999;33 Suppl 5:89–95. [Article in Polish]

How Does Feverfew Quell Migraines?

Once again, I have to admit that we don't quite know. The herb contains a large amount of sesquiterpene lactones, more than half of which are in the form of parthenolide. The parthenolide and other constituents of feverfew are felt to slow the release of serotonin from platelets and certain white blood cells. This, in turn, helps to keep the blood vessels properly toned and reduces the number, length, and severity of migraines. Ingredients in feverfew may also inhibit histamines (which play a role in inflammation), prostaglandin (a substance that plays a role in pain), and arachidonic acid (which is involved in the inflammation process).

Withdrawing Feverfew Leads to an Increase in Migraines

In 1985, the *British Medical Journal* reported on a "reverse" study of feverfew and migraines.[17] Instead of giving the herb to migraineurs, the researchers took it away from some people who already used it.

Seventeen people who ate fresh feverfew leaves daily to prevent migraines were asked to participate in this double-blind, placebo-controlled study. Eight of the volunteers were given capsules with freeze-dried feverfew, while nine were given a placebo. Neither the migraineurs nor the doctors knew who was taking what until the end of the study.

The volunteers getting the feverfew capsules had about the same number of headaches and other side effects, which troubled them about as much as before. That is, the feverfew capsules continued preventing their headaches about as well as the

[17] Johnson ES, Kadam NP, Hylands DM, Hylands, PJ. "Efficacy of feverfew as prophylactic treatment of migraine." *Br Med J (Clin Res Ed)* 1985 Aug 31;291 (6495):569–73.

feverfew leaves had before. But the ones taking the placebo reported a significant increase in the number and severity of headaches, as well as nausea and vomiting. They had almost three times as many migraines as they did before, when they were taking the herb. This study strongly suggests that feverfew can be used prophylactically to prevent migraines from striking.

A Double-Blind, Placebo-Controlled Crossover Study Shows Feverfew Aids in Migraine Prevention

In 1988, British researchers published the results of their randomized, double-blind, placebo-controlled study on feverfew in the prestigious medical journal *Lancet*.[18] Seventy-two volunteers began the study, and fifty-nine were available for full analysis when it was complete.

The study began with a month-long "run-in" period in which the participants were given a placebo and baselines were established. Then they were randomly assigned to either the "feverfew first" group or the "placebo first" group. Those in the "feverfew first" group took one capsule containing 82 mg dried feverfew daily for four months, then took a placebo every day for four months.[19] Those in the "placebo first" group took the placebo first, then the feverfew. Every two months, the participants rated their pain and other symptoms.

The results were gratifying: Treatment with feverfew led to a 24 percent drop in the frequency of attacks, plus a decrease in the nausea and vomiting associated with the migraines.

The researchers broke down the results according to those who had migraines with aura and those without aura. In the sev-

[18] Murphy JJ, Heptinstall S, Mitchell JR. "Randomized double-blind placebo-controlled trial of feverfew in migraine prevention." *Lancet* 1988 July 23;2(8604):189–92.

[19] The feverfew contained about 500 mcg parthenolide.

enteen study participants suffering from migraines with aura, feverfew cut the number of attacks by 32 percent; in the forty-two who had migraines without aura, the number of attacks was reduced by 21 percent. Side effects were mild, mostly nervousness and gastrointestinal disturbance.

Since the quality of feverfew is important, the researchers in this study grew their own to assure that they had a very good product.

A Review of the Feverfew Studies

A 1998 article appearing in the journal *Cephalalgia* reviewed existing studies on feverfew and migraines.[20] The authors analyzed several randomized, placebo-controlled, double-blind studies, trying to arrive at a consensus statement that would sum up the current state of knowledge. Although they did not offer a ringing endorsement of the herb, they reported that of the studies, "the majority favor feverfew over placebo." The side effects reported in the studies "were generally mild and reversible. Mouth ulceration and gastrointestinal symptoms were those most frequently reported." The mouth ulcers appeared primarily in those who chewed the leaves instead of taking capsules. There have also been a few reports of skin problems.

If the majority of studies show that feverfew is better than a placebo for preventing migraines, why don't the study's authors offer a stronger endorsement? After all, isn't that the main criteria for recommending a new drug—that it be better than a placebo? That's true, but the number of studies available for review is small. Medical researchers tend to be cautious. They like to see positive results from many studies conducted by inde-

---

[20] Pittler MH, Vogler BK, Ernst E. "Feverfew as a preventive treatment for migraine: a systematic review." *Cephalalgia* 1998;18:704–8.

pendent researchers at different laboratories in different countries, working under varying conditions, before they pin a blue ribbon on a new substance. In time, I'm sure they'll have what they need to get behind feverfew without reservation. (There's also the issue of feverfew quality, which varies considerably from brand to brand. We'll talk more about that in chapter 5.)

Personally, I have seen a number of patients benefit from taking feverfew. Although only a few of my patients have enjoyed complete relief with the herb, many have reported significant benefits, which is why feverfew is part of my triple therapy.

RIBOFLAVIN FOR MIGRAINES

The final part of my triple therapy is riboflavin. Back in 1994, forty-nine patients suffering from recurrent migraines were given 400 mg of riboflavin every day with breakfast.[21] After the volunteers had been taking the vitamin for at least three months each, they reported fewer migraines (a mean drop of 67 percent in the number of attacks), and less severe attacks (mean improvement was 68 percent). Side effects were minimal: One patient dropped out because of stomach problems. But this study was just a beginning, as it was not double-blind and placebo-controlled.

Fortunately, the same researchers conducted another riboflavin migraine study in 1998.[22] The fifty-five participants in this randomized, placebo-controlled study were given either riboflavin or a placebo for three months. The results indicated

---

[21] Schoenen J, Lenaerts M, Bastings E. "High-dose riboflavin as a prophylactic treatment of migraine: results of an open pilot study." *Cephalalgia* 1994;14:328–29.

[22] Schoenen J, et al. "Effectiveness of high-dose riboflavin in migraine prophylaxis. A randomized controlled trial." *Neurology* 50(2):466–70, 1998.

that the vitamin reduced both the frequency of migraines and the number of days lost to headaches compared to the placebo.

This study answered an interesting question. I had seen many patients try and fail on riboflavin—and my colleagues still tell me that they are not impressed with the efficacy of the vitamin. Why does riboflavin so often get a failing grade? In this study, it took three months of daily riboflavin intake before the researchers saw a difference between the vitamin and a placebo. Most people are not patient enough to take anything for three months before seeing results, so riboflavin doesn't get a chance to work for them. I have no doubt that many patients and doctors tried riboflavin for several weeks then pronounced it a failure, not realizing that had they stayed the course, they might have been rewarded with pain relief.

A FINAL NOTE

The 1996 study with the "wrong" magnesium showed how important it is to use the right form of a nutrient. And the disappointment suffered by many people who have used poor-quality feverfew demonstrates what can happen when inferior substances are used. It's important to make sure you're using the right substances, and to use quality supplements. Always use reputable, high-quality brands of magnesium, riboflavin, and feverfew. (See chapter 5 for a few words on selecting the right feverfew.)

Studies with magnesium, feverfew, and riboflavin are continuing, and researchers are delving deeper into the mysteries of migraines. I have no doubt that in the near future we'll truly understand more about what causes these terrible headaches, and why the triple therapy has helped so many people.

Chapter 5

――◄O►――

Banishing Migraines with the Triple Therapy and More

Magnesium, riboflavin (vitamin B$_2$), and feverfew have worked wonders for many of my patients. By itself, the triple therapy takes a big bite out of migraine frequency, pain, duration, and side effects for many people. But I've found that as good as the triple therapy is, we can go even further by combining it with the other time-tested anti-migraine strategies that make up the Banishing Migraines Program.

This seven-step program for getting rid of migraines combines the best of all worlds: the exciting new and effective triple therapy, sound lifestyle strategies that reduce the risk of migraines, and standard medications when necessary. The seven steps are:

1. Get a proper diagnosis from a medical doctor.
2. Use the triple therapy.
3. Identify and avoid your migraine triggers.
4. Eat to avoid migraines.

5. Take the edge off.
6. Walk it off.
7. Use medicines as necessary.

Before taking any of these steps, see your physician. Tell him or her what you intend to do, ask if it's okay to begin exercising (or change your current regimen), to change your diet, and so on. These seven steps are generally safe, but it's always best to consult with your physician before embarking on any new program.

STEP 1—GET A PROPER DIAGNOSIS FROM A MEDICAL DOCTOR

Headaches strike in many forms, including cluster headaches, tension-type headaches, sinus headaches, organic headaches, temporomandibular joint (TMJ) headaches, migraine headaches, and more. There are also numerous headache subtypes. Among migraineurs, for example, there are those who do and don't get aura, plus people who suffer from the rarer forms of basilar migraine, hemiplegic migraine, ophthalmoplegic migraine, and retinal migraine. Children also suffer from migraines, with and without aura, but the diagnosis is complicated by the fact that they may not have pain, or it may not last as long as it does in adults.

Migraines can be confused with sinus headaches, even by physicians, because the pain may center over the sinuses and be partially relieved by decongestants. Eyestrain headaches can go undiagnosed for some time, while cluster headaches may be initially mistaken for dental problems. The unfortunate truth is that all headaches are not the same. They have different causes and treatments, and prompt different levels of concern. Occasional tension headaches, for example, shouldn't set your health alarm bells ringing. But new and painful headaches may be cause for a great deal of concern, since the pain may herald a serious organic problem such as a brain tumor.

You must know what's wrong before you can begin proper treatment. That's why the program begins with a proper diagnosis from a physician. You want to make sure that you really do have migraine headaches.

Interestingly enough, sometimes just knowing what's wrong can make you feel better. One man, a thirty-five-year-old stockbroker, was suffering from migraines every other month or so. "I'd see a few strange lights, I'd get a little dizzy and nauseous and I'd feel weak. And yes, my head hurt, too. It wasn't that bad, but I thought I was having strokes. It scared the hell out of me because my father died of a stroke in his late thirties. My grandfather also died of a stroke, and two of my uncles had them. It never occurred to me that I was having migraines because I was so focused on strokes. And I was too scared to go to a doctor, because I was sure he would tell me that I had a couple of months to live. The fear was making my life unbearable: Anytime I felt a twinge anywhere in my head, I panicked. Finally, my wife made me go to the doctor, and, I tell you, it's great to know I've only got an occasional migraine. Now that I know what they are, they don't bother me as much."

Remember: Start by getting a proper diagnosis from your medical doctor.

STEP 2—USE THE TRIPLE THERAPY

Magnesium, riboflavin, and feverfew: These three common supplements give the body the tools it needs to fight migraines naturally, effectively, and safely.

Fortunately, it's easy to purchase these three ingredients. You can find them in vitamin and health food stores, in pharmacies, and even in many supermarkets. You can purchase them from catalogs and over the Internet. The supplements are relatively inexpensive. For example, in New York I've found bottles of magnesium for as little as $8, riboflavin for $10, and feverfew for $9. I also checked the prices on the Internet for several well-known companies and found magnesium for $6, riboflavin for $7.50, and feverfew for $6.50.

Using the triple therapy is simple. You take:

- 300–400 mg of magnesium, *plus*
- 400 mg of riboflavin, *plus*
- 100 mg of feverfew

. . . per day. Break your total dosage in half, and take it in two doses per day, with meals.

You can purchase the three members of my triple therapy individually, or combined together in a pill called MigraHealth™. I've had a great deal of experience with this pill, having studied it at my clinic and given it to many patients. In fact, the makers of MigraHealth™ have asked me to consider being a spokesman for the product. (You can get MigraHealth™ (also sold as MigraLief®) in major grocery, drug, and discount stores, as well as on the Internet.) If you're using MigraHealth™ or a similar formulation that combines all three in the right amounts, you can take one pill twice a day, each with a meal.

Calcium and magnesium compete to be absorbed in the body, so if you are taking calcium supplements, it's best not to take the calcium pill at the same time you're taking the triple therapy. Take the calcium a couple hours before or after taking the magnesium-riboflavin-feverfew combination.

Because magnesium and riboflavin are well-known substances that have long been manufactured by various companies, we don't have to worry too much about being let down by inferior materials. If you purchase your products from a reputable company, you should be getting the real thing. However, be sure to read the labels carefully. Magnesium, for example, comes in different forms. You want to make sure you're taking magnesium oxide or chelated magnesium. If one type causes diarrhea or stomach pain, as it may in some people, you might have to try the other.

Unfortunately, selecting the right brand of feverfew can be difficult, for one brand is not necessarily identical to another. Like all herbs, feverfew is a living plant shaped by its environment; the soil, climate, and so forth.

Imagine oranges growing in two different orchards. The first orchard is in the middle of prime farmland, so the oranges get plenty of sunlight and water, and send their roots down into rich soil. The other orchard is in a desertlike area with poor soil, right next to a major highway. These oranges must be doused with fertilizers and chemicals to keep them alive, and their growth is stunted by lack of water and exposure to car exhaust. Clearly, the oranges grown in the two orchards are going to taste different, and have different amounts of nutrients. The same is true with feverfew. As with all herbs, feverfew's makeup changes with the soil, climate, pollution, and other factors.

The differences don't stop there, for processing can introduce new variations. Suppose there are two different factories turning oranges into orange juice. They start with oranges from the same orchard, but have different procedures. One factory makes a "rough" orange juice, leaving in the pulp and perhaps a few pits as well. The other factory produces a "refined" drink, straining the juice over and over again to remove every single bit of pulp and every single pit, then heating it to high temperatures to homogenize it, and adding calcium.

Processing can change feverfew even more than it does orange juice, for there's no definitive agreement on what constitutes feverfew. You see, there isn't one thing that gives the feverfew plant its "feverfewness," for the feverfew plant contains hundreds of different chemicals. We don't really know which ones have the most health benefits, or even which ones are absolutely necessary to make feverfew "work."

There is no agreement on which of many substances is most "feverfewish," so manufacturers will focus on different chemicals to make their extracts. For example, one manufacturer may extract substances 1, 2, 5, 7, and 9; another may extract 1, 3, 4, 8, and 9; a third may select 2, 3, 5, 8, and 11. They're all feverfew, but one may contain the "antimigraine ingredient" and another may not. Since we don't know exactly which ingredient or ingredients quell migraines, we can't say that this brand of feverfew is better than another—unless we study each brand individually.

And that's the key to finding the right brand of feverfew—clinical studies. You want a brand of feverfew that has been tested and found to reduce migraines. All manufacturers will claim that feverfew relieves migraines, but you want a brand that is *identical to the brand used in the testing.* How will you know if the feverfew you are purchasing is the same feverfew used in the studies? The manufacturer will say so, on the bottle label or the supporting advertising. Remember: All manufacturers will tell you that feverfew is good for headaches. You want the brand that specifically says it is the *same thing* that was used in the successful studies.

Once you begin taking the triple therapy, be patient. It takes a month or two to see the full benefits from magnesium and feverfew, while up to three months may pass before you notice benefits from riboflavin.

Finally, the question all my patients eventually ask: How long will I need to take the three supplements? Probably for a long time. Remember, it's likely that you're suffering from migraines because you have chronically low levels of magnesium, and possibly riboflavin as well. Perhaps you're not getting enough from your diet, or maybe your need is greater because of stress or other factors. Or it might be that you're taking in enough but your body doesn't handle these nutrients well. For whatever reason, you need to replace what's been missing—and to keep on replacing it. It's very difficult to do this by diet alone, especially if you're not absorbing nutrients well, if the calcium in your diet is competing with the magnesium for absorption and so forth. Eating a health-enhancing diet with magnesium- and riboflavin-rich foods is certainly a good idea. And changing your lifestyle—reducing your stress, increasing your exercise, avoiding migraine triggers, etc.—reducing what is perhaps an elevated need for the nutrients is also helpful. Most people, however, can expect to continue to take the supplements for many years.

Don't forget, however, that the propensity toward migraines lessens with advancing age. As you grow older, or ladies, as you pass through menopause, your need for the supplements may fade, or might even disappear entirely.

The Odds Are Slim, But . . .

It's remarkably difficult to overdose on riboflavin, for if you ingest too much, the body excretes the excess through the urine. The vitamin will give a bright yellow coloration to the urine: Don't worry, it's not harmful.

However, it is possible to take in too much magnesium. This is unlikely, especially if you take the amounts recommended in the program, but it's possible. The kidneys are responsible for excreting any magnesium surplus, so kidney disease or failure may allow levels of the mineral to build to dangerous amounts. The elderly, who may suffer from reduced kidney function, can also slowly develop magnesium excess.

The signs and symptoms of too much magnesium include drowsiness, breathing difficulty, weakness, and lethargy. And since magnesium "opposes" the mineral calcium in your body, excessive amounts of it can cause symptoms of calcium deficiency.

Feverfew can interfere with the normal ability of the blood to clot. If you're taking any anticoagulant medications, or have any blood problems, be sure to discuss your use of feverfew with your physician. And beware of chewing feverfew leaves (rather than taking pills), as doing so may cause ulcers in the mouth.

As with anything involving the use of supplements, diets, and changes in habits, you should discuss this program with your physician before beginning it. This is especially true for pregnant or nursing women.

Magnesium, riboflavin, and feverfew anchor the Banishing Migraines Program, but they're only one of seven parts. For best results, it is important to put the entire program into practice.

STEP 3—IDENTIFY AND AVOID YOUR MIGRAINE TRIGGERS

We don't know exactly why migraineurs are susceptible to the terrible headaches and associated symptoms, and we can't identify a gene or group of genes that causes the problem. But this much we do know: Millions of susceptible people have a propensity toward migraines, and migraine triggers often set them off.

The triggers can be almost anything, including common foods such as cheese, bacon, nuts, avocados, chocolate, yeast, spices, hot dogs, corn, anything fermented, red wine, and beverages containing caffeine. Other triggers include missing a meal, stress, fatigue, bright lights, certain medicines or odors, air pollution, changes in the weather, and changes in hormones.

There are hundreds of potential triggers, ranging from common to rare, from physical items to situations. They're at work, at home; they may be on your plate, on your spouse's skin, or in your medicine; they may be obvious or subtle; easy to avoid or omnipresent.

One way to reduce the number of migraines you get is to learn how to identify those triggers, then avoid them. That's all it took for one physician to eliminate his migraines. Back in the 1960s and 1970s, this doctor, a "specialist's specialist," used to go to several different hospitals handling the most difficult cases. His life was high-stress because he was dealing with many very ill patients, and he was often called away from bed in the middle of the night to attend to them, but he loved his job. The only problem was the splitting migraines he kept getting.

"It was bad," he explained. "The pain was incredible. And the nausea—it was all I could do to keep my mind focused while I was seeing the patients and talking to their doctors. Finally I realized that the migraines always hit me on the days I went to a certain hospital. The place was terrible! The owners had cut back on everything, the place was understaffed, poorly equipped, poorly maintained. I was always fighting with the administrator, trying to get better care for my patients. And the whole time I was there, I'd be gulping coffee. I finally realized that going to that hospital was making me sick! So I just stopped going. I told the doctors I worked with to put their difficult cases in a different hospital, and I saw them there. Between not going to that one hospital and not gulping down gallons of coffee, my migraines went away. Absolutely gone."

You'll learn how to recognize triggers, how to track your migraines and other symptoms, and how to avoid many of the things that may be making you hurt so much, in chapters 6 and 7. Finding out what sets off your migraines, then avoiding the trigger(s), may be all the "medicine" you need. And if that doesn't completely eliminate your headaches, there's a good chance it will at least cut back on the number of attacks.

STEP 4—EAT TO AVOID MIGRAINES

"I was getting these incredible headaches for about two years," Bob, an executive in his thirties, explained. "I suffered for several months, then I finally went to my internist, who said I had migraines and gave me a prescription for some medicine. The medicine didn't help much, so I went back to the doctor. This time he sent me to a neurologist, who gave me a different drug. That was better, but still didn't solve the problem, so we tried another drug, then another. The situation was pretty bad.

"Then I happened to go back East to visit my cousin. We were casually talking about this and that, catching up. He asked me when I started getting the migraines and I said, 'Two years ago, when the new owners took over the company.'

"And then it hit me: My migraines started when the new owners came in and started ordering in these cheese plates with exotic cheeses for the executives a couple times a week. I never ate much cheese before, and then only standard cheeses like Jack or American. I stopped eating the exotic cheese and bingo! No more headaches!

"After being migraine-free for a few months I started experimenting and figured out it was the Swiss Gruyère cheese."

An incredible variety of foods can trigger migraines, but that's not to say that they "cause" the headaches. Do you remember the story of King Arthur of Camelot? According to the legend, a large stone with a beautiful sword set in it appeared in the forest. All the famous and lesser-known knights tried to remove the sword from the stone, but it remained stuck fast. No one could budge it. Then one day young Arthur, still a boy, pulled the sword from the stone. He, and only he, could handle the magnificent weapon.

Think of the sword as your migraine, and Arthur as the food that triggers the headache. Unless the right food comes along, your migraine/sword will sit in the stone forever, causing you no trouble. But if the Arthur/food is present, even if it's a small quantity of an otherwise innocent food, the sword will be unsheathed.

We don't know how many migraines are caused by food triggers, but the estimates run quite high. Many people are able to significantly reduce their migraine problem simply by changing their diets.

Identifying the food trigger can be difficult, for we tend to eat many different kinds of foods, and often don't know all of the ingredients in the meals we eat at restaurants, or in the numerous canned and packaged foods we consume. It's well worth the effort, however, to take the time to figure it out.

You'll learn how to identify and avoid food triggers in chapter 6—plus how to avoid foods that encourage inflammation, and how to get plenty of magnesium and riboflavin in your daily diet.

STEP 5—TAKE THE EDGE OFF

"I live in fear," says twenty-eight-year-old Kelly. "When my migraine prodrome starts, I freak out because I know the pain is coming next. When the pain and nausea start, I panic. Then, once the migraine is fully gone I live in fear for several days, waiting for the next one to hit.

"Do you know about the sword of Damocles, the one that was held up over the guy's head by just a single hair? That's how I feel with my migraines: The hair that holds the sword up is always about to break, and that sword is going to start cutting through my head. I'm afraid of everything. I avoid problems because I think stress will set off a migraine. I only eat certain foods and never eat out because I'm afraid some food will trigger the next migraine. I get panicked if I smell any perfume or other odors. It's a terrible way to live."

Fear, anxiety, depression, panic, feelings of helplessness and hopelessness; these are all common "side effects" of migraines. That's bad enough, but it gets even worse when you consider that these negative feelings can have triggerlike effects, making the migraine problem even worse. We can't say for certain, but it's a good bet that Kelly's fear is contributing to her migraines— perhaps making them strike more often, hurt more, or last longer than they might otherwise.

Taking the edge off your stress and negative feelings is an important part of the overall plan for relieving migraines and their side effects. You'll be introduced to some simple techniques for taking the edge off in chapter 8.

STEP 6—WALK IT OFF

Exercise is not a cure for migraines, but it does strengthen overall health and help relieve the stress that can contribute to the problem. I recommend all kinds of exercise: aerobic, strengthening, stretching, group, individual, organized, free-form. It really doesn't matter what type you choose, as long as it builds health and relieves stress, you do it regularly and properly, and you *have fun.*

"Having fun is the key," said twenty-five-year-old Krista. "My doctor told me to exercise to reduce my stress, so I *really* exercised. I set up a program of aerobics, weights, and stretching. I got a stopwatch, a clipboard, a paper and pen, and I *really* went at it. Every single day at exactly the same time I did exactly the right amount of exercise, the exact number of repetitions, the exact number of minutes of aerobics. I was an exercising machine! It was driving me crazy, trying to be so perfect! It was making me even *more* stressed. Finally I tossed out my clipboard and stopwatch, and stopped trying to be great. Now I just have fun."

We'll talk more about exercise in chapter 9.

STEP 7—USE MEDICINES AS NECESSARY

The last of the seven steps is to use standard medications as necessary. There are a host of such medicines, including Imitrex, Maxalt, Zomig, Inderal, Depakote, Midrin, aspirin, and more. It's true that every single drug has side effects, sometimes serious ones such as stomach upset, weakness, elevated or low blood pressure, rapid heartbeat, and chest pain. The goal is to wean yourself away from these drugs via the triple therapy and the rest of the program. But sometimes medicines are necessary. It may take several weeks or a few months for the full effect of the program to kick in, or you may have an occasional migraine that has to be taken care of, right now.

In chapter 10 we'll review the pros and cons of the various drugs prescribed for migraines. You'll learn what each drug is expected to do, how well it works, and what to watch for when using it.

REMEMBER: ALL SEVEN STEPS
ARE IMPORTANT

That's the seven-step Banishing Migraines Program: Get a proper diagnosis from a medical doctor, use the triple therapy, identify and avoid your migraine triggers, eat to avoid migraines, take the edge off, walk it off, and use medicines as necessary. Any one step may make a significant dent in your migraine problem. In fact, many people are helped by the triple therapy alone. But I must emphasize that *it's best to follow the entire program.* Remember, migraines are more than just a headache plus some other symptoms. Migraines are a syndrome, a whole-body phenomenon that must be met with a comprehensive program involving body, mind, and emotions on many levels. The good news is that you *can* do it: I've seen many people banish their migraines just this way.

A VITAL EXTRA STEP

Discuss my triple therapy and Banishing Migraines Program with your physician. He or she should know that you're going to be taking magnesium, riboflavin, and feverfew supplements, how often and in what amount. Tell your doctor about any dietary changes you intend to make, and have a checkup to make sure that it's safe to begin or change your exercise regimen.

Chapter 6

━━━━━━━━━◀O▶━━━━━━━━━

Eating to Avoid Migraines

- Do you enjoy a glass of red wine now and then?
- Is scotch, brandy, bourbon, or champagne "your drink"?
- Are you a "chocoholic"?
- Do you adore creamy blue cheese salad dressing or a good, sharp cheddar cheese?
- Does freshly baked yeast bread set your mouth to watering?
- Do you enjoy good pungent sauerkraut or mouth-puckering pickled herring?
- Do you drink more than two cups of coffee, tea, or soft drinks per day?
- Do you eat packaged or prepared foods regularly?
- Are you a Chinese food freak?
- Do you eat potato chips, dips, frozen pizza, processed meats, or canned soups?
- Do you love ham, hot dogs, luncheon meat, or sausage?

- Do you fast, diet, skip meals, or eat high-sugar foods as snacks?

If you said yes to even one item, your migraines may be triggered by foods. In other words, you may be eating yourself sick.

IS FOOD TO BE FEARED?

"One man's meat is another man's poison." Migraineurs know very well that this old English proverb is all too true. For me, a glass of wine is the perfect accompaniment to a delightful dinner. For you, perhaps, the same few ounces of wine are an invitation to disaster. Or maybe chocolate fudge cake is your particular poison, if not a fine Stilton cheese.

Many migraine sufferers find themselves on the road to yet another headache after eating certain *trigger foods,* which usually contain one or more of the following:

- alcohol
- amines
- caffeine
- food additives (MSG, nitrites, aspartame)

The foods we eat are at least partly responsible for the significant increase in migraines in the past ten years that's left us cringing in pain. That's because, in addition to the alcohol, amines, and caffeine, our foods contain more chemicals, pesticides, herbicides, preservatives, and other additives than ever before. We consume more fast foods, processed foods, frozen foods, and preserved foods than any population in history, and all of these contain plentiful amounts of additives with migraine-causing potential.

A bewildering variety of things that we eat and drink can trigger migraines. But they all have one thing in common: They cause blood vessels in the brain to dilate and become inflamed. Some substances found in foods, such as *nitrites* (the major preservatives found in cured meats, hot dogs, bacon, and ham), are powerful vasodilators that go straight to work stretching out the blood vessels. Others, like the amino acid *tyramine,* the flavor enhancer *MSG* (often disguised on the labels as "natural flavoring" and other euphemisms), and everybody's favorite additive, *caffeine,* constrict the blood vessels at first, but can end up triggering excessive dilation later on. Still others, like *alcohol,* initially cause blood vessel dilation, followed by constriction, followed by more dilation—a case of blood vessel "twitchiness" that results in that awful throbbing sensation in your head.

Although the list of foods, drinks, and food additives that may cause migraines is a long one, *nobody* gets a migraine from all of them. Some people may only be sensitive to chocolate, for example, or to certain combinations of foods: maybe a bacon cheeseburger. Others may be able to eat small amounts of an offending food (one orange, for example), but develop crushing migraines if they exceed a certain threshold (three oranges). To make matters more complicated, some foods may trigger a migraine some of the time but not always. This may have something to do with the stress load exerted on the nervous system at the time. High stress levels increase the chances of dietary sensitivities, which means you might be able to get away with eating a trigger food when things are otherwise calm and stress-free. But if you're under the gun, watch out!

The only way to know for sure whether or not a food, drink, or food additive triggers your migraines is to eliminate the suspected item from your diet completely, then slowly reintroduce it and watch for reactions. But before we get into the elimination diet, let's take a closer look at the four major dietary triggers of migraine headaches, and the foods and drinks they inhabit.

Dietary Trigger #1: Alcohol

One look at the bloodshot eyes and ruddy cheeks of a heavy drinker and you know that alcohol is a powerful vasodilator—at least initially. This widening of the blood vessels can set the wheels of a migraine in motion, causing the body to respond by clamping down on them. The blood vessels may respond to that by widening, then constricting, then widening again. (Oh, that pounding in your head!) Or they may simply settle into the constriction mode. Either way, the result of alcohol ingestion is the constriction of blood vessels. For those who have a tendency toward migraines, even a couple of sips of alcohol can bring on an attack.

Many kinds of alcohol also contain additives and preservatives such as sulfites and tyramine that bring about headaches by inducing blood vessel changes. Red wine, which contains both of these substances, is the most likely offender, but other dark-colored alcoholic drinks are also common headache triggers.

Then there's the hangover headache, a painful side effect of alcohol consumption that is brought on by a different mechanism than migraines. Surprisingly, it's the impurities in the liquor, rather than the liquor itself, that are usually the culprits.

So ingestion of alcohol can deliver a triple whammy to headache sufferers: through blood vessel changes instigated by the alcohol itself, or through its additives, or through hangovers. Is it any wonder that alcohol usually tops the list of things to avoid for prevention of migraines?

Alcoholic Drinks Most Likely to Cause Migraines

It's best to avoid alcohol completely if you suffer from migraines, especially these popular drinks:

* red wine
* brandy
* scotch
* bourbon
* champagne
* beer, particularly the darker-colored brews

Alcoholic Drinks Least Likely to Cause Migraines

Some people can get away with drinking small amounts of the following, but when stress levels are high or other headache inducers are present, even these may bring on a migraine:

* clear liquor, like vodka
* white wine

Dietary Trigger #2: Amines

Back in high school chemistry, we all learned that amino acids are the building blocks of protein. But amino acids are not the most basic protein substances, for they too are made up of smaller substances called amines. Certain amines are notorious migraine inducers, triggering the release of hormones that constrict the blood vessels. The blood vessels respond by dilating, and the familiar throbbing begins. Amines can also activate certain neurotransmitters that set off a migraine attack. The most common perpetrator is *tyramine,* an important ingredient in adrenaline, which causes an estimated 25 percent of all migraine headaches. Many people find that simply consuming a tyramine-free diet is enough to relieve their migraines.

An amine found primarily in chocolate, called *phenylethyl-amine* (PEA), has similar effects on the blood vessels. It's no surprise that the world is loaded with chocolate lovers, for PEA is the same chemical that's released in our bodies when we fall in love. It's a natural mood elevator, a stress reliever, and can even help enhance memory. Unfortunately, PEA can also bring on a killer headache—turning this mood elevator into a guaranteed mood deflator!

Foods Containing Tyramine

To see if tyramine is your migraine trigger, eliminate the following foods from your diet and watch what happens. Granted, the list is long, but you'll probably be able to resume eating many (if not most) of these foods once you've eliminated them as the cause of your headaches.

Aged cheese (listed in order of highest amount of tyramine):

- English Stilton
- blue cheese
- sharp cheddar
- Danish blue
- mozzarella
- Swiss Gruyère
- feta
- Parmesan
- Gorgonzola

Other tyramine-containing foods that may give you trouble:

- aged and cured meats such as bacon, ham, hot dogs, and sausage, and game meats such as venison
- avocados
- bananas
- bean pods
- beer and ale
- broad beans
- buttermilk
- cabbage
- cream
- eggplant
- fermented foods
- figs
- fish, pickled or preserved (caviar included)
- Italian beans
- lentils
- lima beans
- liver, especially chicken liver, and other organ meats
- navy beans
- nuts (including peanut butter or other nut butter)
- onions
- peas
- pickled herring
- pineapple
- pinto beans
- raisins
- red wine
- salad dressings
- sauerkraut
- seeds (sunflower, pumpkin, sesame)
- snow peas

- sour cream
- soybeans
- soy sauce
- spinach
- tomatoes
- vinegar and foods containing vinegar (catsup, relish, mayonnaise, mustard, etc.)
- yeast products (freshly baked bread or cake; foods containing yeast extract, such as bouillon, soup mix, etc.)
- yogurt

Foods Containing Phenylethylamine

Be wary of these PEA-containing foods:

- chocolate
- aspartame (NutraSweet)

Keep in mind that not all of these foods will trigger a migraine in any one individual. The trick is to find out which ones do, then avoid them.

Dietary Trigger #3: Caffeine

Caffeine is a painkiller and a vasoconstrictor, so it can actually help ease the pain of a migraine when blood vessels become dilated. It is, in fact, one of the major ingredients in certain migraine medications. But you can end up doing more harm than good if you overindulge in caffeine and it causes overconstriction of the blood vessels.

Daily overuse of caffeine is a common problem. Those who consume more than two cups of coffee or two cans of soft drinks daily (about 150–250 mg of caffeine), or an equivalent amount of caffeine through prescription or nonprescription drugs, can find themselves relying on caffeine to keep their blood vessels from dilating unnaturally. But then, if their caffeine intake suddenly decreases, the blood vessels can widen and a migraine may strike. This is known as a *rebound headache,* the scourge of many a worker who drinks several cups of coffee at work but not much (if any) during time away from work. Headaches that occur in the early morning before that first cup of coffee and "weekend migraines" are often the result of an initial overindulgence followed by a drastic drop in caffeine consumption.

To make matters worse, caffeine (like many drugs) becomes less and less effective over time as the body builds up a tolerance. So you may find yourself drinking more and more coffee or cola or popping more and more medication to keep headaches at bay.

Bad as that sounds, there's more to come. Caffeine can also interfere with normal sleep patterns, or just plain rob you of sleep, and the lack of sleep can set the stage for another headpounder. Daily consumption of large amounts of caffeine can also make you more anxious and depressed. A recent study published in the *New England Journal of Medicine* showed that caffeine also increases the risk of a miscarriage. For all of these reasons, I urge my patients to cut back or completely eliminate caffeine from their diets. Obviously, if your body is used to a high intake of caffeine, it's not a good idea to stop cold turkey. Begin by cutting out one cup of coffee, soda, or caffeine-containing medication each day for a week. Then reduce a little more the following week, and continue until your diet is caffeine-free. You may need to stay at one level for more than a week to avoid a caffeine-withdrawal headache. That's fine; the important thing is to keep cutting back, even if only very gradually. Remember that this is an ongoing process, not a race—although some of my patients prefer to stop caffeine all at once, suffer for a day or two (I give them medication to cope with withdrawal headaches), and get it over with. It is especially appropriate for people whose headaches become very severe even if they eliminate one cup at a time, thus prolonging their agony.

Foods and Drinks Containing Caffeine

- coffee (especially the kind made by drip coffeemakers)
- tea (especially black, oolong, mint, and Chinese green)
- soft drinks (such as Coca-Cola, Diet Coke, Dr. Pepper, Mountain Dew, Pepsi-Cola, Diet Pepsi, Sunkist Orange)
- chocolate (including milk chocolate)
- cocoa

Instead of the drinks listed above, try decaffeinated coffee, tea, and soft drinks, light-colored soft drinks like ginger ale or Seven-Up, sparkling water—or just plain water, one of the best drinks in the universe.

Some Nonprescription (Over-the-Counter) Drugs Containing Caffeine

- Anacin—for pain
- Dexatrim—a weight-loss aid
- Excedrin—for pain
- Excedrin Migraine—for migraine
- Midol—to ease menstrual cramps
- NoDoz—to help you stay awake
- Vanquish—for headache pain
- Vivarin—to help you stay awake

Some Prescription Drugs Containing Caffeine

- Cafergot—used for migraines and other headaches.
- Darvon Compound-65—a mild narcotic painkiller used for mild to moderate pain.
- Fioricet—a powerful barbiturate, used for tension headaches. This non-narcotic is also packaged under the brand names of Anolor 300, Esgic, and Esgic-Plus.
- Fiorinal—a powerful barbiturate, used for tension headaches. This non-narcotic is also packaged under the name Isollyl.
- Fiorinal with Codeine—a narcotic painkiller and barbiturate, used for tension headaches.
- Norgesic—for relief of mild to moderate pain due to muscle disorders. Also packaged under the name Norgesic Forte.
- Synalgos-DC—a narcotic painkiller used for moderate to moderately severe pain.

You'll also find caffeine in Amaphen, Anoquan, Aspirin compound with codeine, Aspirin-Free Bayer Select, Aspirin Free Excedrin, Cafermine, Cafetrate, Caffedrine, Dexitac, Dristan AF, Fendol, Histosal, Kolephrin, Lanorinal, Pacaps Compound, Darvon Compound, Quick Pep, Saleto-D, Sinapils, Supac, and Wigraine, among others. Be sure to check the package for full details on any medication you take.

And watch out for a popular Brazilian herb called guarana, used to increase energy. It's loaded with caffeine.

Dietary Trigger #4: Food Additives

Of the many additives in our foods today, the two most likely to trigger migraines are *MSG* (monosodium glutamate) and *nitrites*.

You may remember the big MSG scare that swept across the country a couple of decades ago. Suddenly we began hearing about how this flavor enhancer, widely used in Chinese food, was causing terrible headaches. Naturally, the media had over-hyped the scare, but once things died down a bit, we realized that MSG is a vasoconstrictor that can initiate migraines—that is, in certain people.

Besides Chinese food, you'll find MSG in meat tenderizer (Accent) and a great many packaged and prepared foods. But even though MSG is usually found in packaged (and therefore, labeled) foods, its presence isn't always obvious. Watch for the words "hydrolyzed protein," "autolyzed yeast," "sodium caseinate," "yeast extract," "hydrolized oat flour," "texturized protein," or "calcium caseinate"—words that food manufacturers use to quietly announce the presence of MSG without spelling it out.

Foods Containing MSG

- Accent brand seasoning
- bacon bits
- bouillon
- breaded foods
- canned meat
- Chinese food
- dips
- dry-roasted peanuts
- frozen dinners
- frozen pizza
- frozen pot pies
- gelatin
- potato chips, corn chips

- processed cheese
- processed meats
- salad dressing
- seasoning
- soup—canned, dried, or frozen
- soy sauce
- stuffing

As with MSG, there was also a nitrite scare many years ago, with articles in major newspapers and magazines warning us that nitrites (or a different form called nitrates) may cause cancer. Nitrites are preservatives added to cured meats (bologna, hot dogs, smoked meats, bacon, ham) to give them their nice pink color. But nitrites are not confined to meat products alone: They're also found in food colorings and vegetables in brine! Although the jury is still out on nitrites as carcinogens, they do act as strong vasodilators that can instigate migraines. Check the labels on your packaged foods for "sodium nitrite," "sodium nitrate," "potassium nitrite," or "potassium nitrate." These are all ways of saying that nitrites are present.

Unfortunately, not all foods that contain nitrites are labeled. For example, the fruits and vegetables in salad bars or grocery stores are sometimes sprayed with nitrites to preserve their appearance or freshness. (Check with the management before buying.)

MSG and nitrites are widespread, so if they bother you, you will probably have to give up several foods, then clean out your kitchen cupboards, refrigerator, and freezer pretty thoroughly to rid yourself of these chemicals.

Foods Containing Nitrites

- bacon
- bratwurst
- beef jerky
- corn dogs
- corned beef
- food coloring agent FD&C yellow #5
- ham
- hot dogs
- luncheon meats, including those made from turkey
- liverwurst
- meat tenderizers
- pastrami
- pork and beans
- salami
- sausage
- smoked fish
- Spam
- vegetables in brine

ARE YOU ALLERGIC, INTOLERANT, OR JUST PLAIN SENSITIVE?

Although it's a relatively rare phenomenon, a migraine may be a response to a hypersensitivity to certain foods. Notice that I said a "food hypersensitivity," not an allergy. A true food allergy (which probably exists in only a small percentage of the population who are allergic to things such as peanuts or shellfish) incites your body's immune system to act as if it's being attacked. Responding to imaginary enemies, the immune system can unleash a full-blown defensive, causing the throat to swell up, making breathing difficult, setting the heart pounding wildly, triggering skin rashes or hives, and so forth. With a true food allergy, you may only have to take a bite or two of the offending food to bring on these symptoms, which can also include nausea, vomiting, diarrhea, tremors, asthma attacks, fatigue, and headaches. Severe cases of food allergy can even result in a life-threatening reaction known as *anaphylactic shock.*

Much more often, however, the offending food triggers a *food intolerance,* a much milder reaction that can cause digestive problems such as bloating, diarrhea or constipation, nasal congestion, or headaches. These symptoms are annoying, but not life-threatening. The "danger threshold" for the offending food is usually much higher in food intolerance than it is in food allergy. In other words, you may have to eat a lot of that food before you get a reaction. And should you develop a headache in response to a food intolerance, it will most likely be a by-product of the nasal or sinus congestion produced by the intolerance, rather than a reaction to the food itself. These headaches are usually more of a reaction to the reaction, in a sense.

A *food sensitivity* is a heightened reaction to a substance, but the reaction doesn't seem to involve the immune system. These are usually found in those who are very sensitive to low levels of environmental toxins: In other words, a lot of things bother them, possibly because of a combination of enzyme deficiencies and a certain amount of central nervous system damage.

Whatever the reason, the foods and food additives that may cause sensitivity, intolerance, or allergy include:

- alcoholic beverages
- apples
- beef
- benzoic acid
- caffeine

- cheese
- chocolate*
- citrus fruits*
- corn and corn products
- dairy products*
- eggs*
- fish
- food additives and preservatives
- goat's milk
- grapes
- processed meat, meat products
- nightshade plants (eggplant, peppers, potatoes, tomatoes)
- oats
- onions
- peanuts
- pork
- rye
- shellfish
- soy and soy products
- sugar
- tartrazine
- tomatoes
- tree nuts (walnuts, pecans, etc.)
- wheat and wheat products*
- yeast

LOW BLOOD SUGAR AND HEADACHES

Another common cause of headaches is low blood sugar (hypo-glycemia). If you've ever skipped a meal (and who hasn't?),

*Foods most likely to induce hypersensitivity-related migraines.

fasted, or simply waited too long to eat, you're familiar with the weak, tired, headachey feeling that washes over you when your glucose levels dip too low. You may have also felt like this after eating a sugary snack on an empty stomach. With nothing else to slow its entrance into your bloodstream, the sugar prompted a sudden rise in blood sugar. Insulin was then released to bring the levels back down to normal. But sometimes too much insulin is released and "eats up" too much blood sugar, pushing the levels of this internal fuel down too low, leaving you dizzy, shaky, light-headed, and probably on the brink of a headache.

Hypoglycemia is fairly easy to avoid. All you need to do is make sure you eat small, balanced meals several times a day, while avoiding high-sugar foods. You may need to make a point of keeping your blood sugar levels fairly even by eating three meals and three snacks a day—one midmorning, one midafternoon, and one at bedtime. Or perhaps you'd rather eat six *small* meals a day, maybe one every three hours. Either way, make sure you have some protein at each meal or snack (a small amount of cottage cheese, meat, poultry, fish, or eggs, depending on which foods don't set off your migraines), and some complex carbohydrates (fresh fruit, vegetables, whole grains, etc.). Reduce or avoid the consumption of simple carbohydrates (sugar, honey, candy, etc.), especially when taken alone. Fruit should always be consumed with a small amount of protein, which will slow the entrance of its sugar (fructose) into the bloodstream, preventing a blood sugar spike.

WHAT *SHOULD* YOU EAT?

Can you see a pattern emerging here? Food-wise, it's primarily the processed, packaged, sugary, unnatural foods that bring on migraine headaches. That's why it makes sense to eat the most healthful and natural diet possible: Not only will doing so prevent hypersensitivity, it will also bolster your overall health. Stick with fresh (unsprayed, organic) fruits and vegetables; whole grains (rice, if you tend toward food allergies); fresh fish, meats, or poultry; fruit juice, herbal tea, and water, and you'll most likely have fewer headaches and better health overall. It's also a good idea to include foods that are rich in the following (unless these foods happen to be triggers for you):

- *Copper.* This mineral helps to release iron from storage and affects the strength and function of the blood vessels. A deficiency of copper is associated with high blood pressure. Copper is found primarily in seafood, liver, whole grains, legumes, nuts, seeds, and cocoa.
- *Folic acid.* This vitamin helps to ensure that the blood is well oxygenated. Getting adequate amounts of folic acid is important, for a shortfall of oxygen to the brain can bring on headaches. Folic acid is present in large amounts in green leafy vegetables, organ meats, beans, peanuts, oranges, and sprouts.
- *Iron.* Known for its important role in the oxygenation of the blood, this mineral also plays a part in synthesizing serotonin, the "feel-good" hormone. Too little iron increases the risk of headaches and other kinds of pain, as well as fatigue, poor temperature regulation, and a compromised immune status. The best sources of iron are foods that come from animals, such as oysters, liver, clams, and red meat. Other sources include enriched grain products, spinach, peas, legumes, plus acidic foods like tomato sauce that are cooked for extended periods of time in iron pots or cast-iron frying pans. (The food absorbs the iron.) Be careful about taking in too much iron, for excessive amounts have been implicated in higher rates of coronary artery disease. This is more of a

problem for men than for menstruating women, who lose iron with their menstrual blood.

- *Magnesium.* This mineral is, of course, one part of the triple therapy. A deficiency results in vasoconstriction and contributes to inflammation of the nerves, which can equal headache pain. Good sources of magnesium include wheat bran, green vegetables, legumes, and nuts.
- *L-tryptophan.* The development of migraines may be due in part to a deficiency in the brain hormone serotonin. L-tryptophan is the dietary substance from which serotonin is made, so adding lots of this amino acid to your diet may help raise your resistance to future attacks. Good sources of L-tryptophan include milk, turkey, and carbohydrates.
- *Niacin.* Often called vitamin B_3, niacin helps increase blood flow to the brain and reduce vasoconstriction. Deficiencies of niacin are known to contribute to headaches. Good sources include fish, chicken, wheat bran, mushrooms, asparagus, peanuts, and enriched breads and cereals.
- *Omega-3 fatty acids.* Found primarily in cold-water fish and fish oil, as well as in green vegetables and certain plant oils, the omega-3 fatty acids help reduce the inflammation response that contributes to the migraine process. The resultant swelling and pain of blood vessels in the head and face may be eased in part by eating the following foods on a regular basis: salmon, mackerel, albacore tuna, herring, sardines, lake trout, Atlantic sturgeon, flaxseed, walnuts, canola oil, and leafy green vegetables. Don't overconsume fish oil or fish oil capsules, though, as they can interfere with the proper clotting of the blood.
- *Linolenic and linoleic acid.* The body produces substances called *prostaglandins* in response to injury, and they play a part in bringing about inflammation. But *alpha-linolenic acid* (ALA), which is found in green vegetables and certain

other plants, can help block prostaglandin production. *Gamma-linolenic acid* (GLA), found in evening primrose oil, borage seed oil, and blackcurrant oil, helps prevent blood platelets from clumping together, improving the circulation and reducing inflammation. And *linoleic acid,* which is found in certain light vegetable oils such as corn, soybean, safflower, and sunflower oils, also helps hinder the production of prostaglandins. So to help control inflammation, consider adding green vegetables and one or more of these plant oils to your diet.

- *Riboflavin.* This vitamin, also called B$_2$, is a part of the triple therapy. It's an important ingredient in the production of cellular energy, and researchers have noticed that the mitochondrial energy reserve drops between migraine attacks. We suspect that riboflavin can help keep the energy levels up, thus reducing migraines. Good sources of riboflavin include milk, mushrooms, liver, spinach, and enriched grains.

THE ELIMINATION DIET

In order to determine the trigger foods that might be setting off your migraines, it's necessary to eat the blandest, least allergenic diet possible, then slowly add suspected trigger foods one at a time, while watching for reactions. This can be a long, tedious process, but it may be necessary if foods or food additives are the cause of your attacks.

To begin the process, rid your diet of additives, preservatives, caffeine, and alcohol. That's tougher than it sounds, leaving you with a diet based on easily tolerated foods such as brown rice, fresh vegetables, fresh fruit (except citrus), and lightly cooked fish or chicken. Unprocessed fruit and vegetable juice is also fine (invest in a juicer and make it yourself!), as are herbal teas and lots of water (at least eight glasses a day). If you like dressing on your salad, use preservative-free canola oil mixed with herbs and a little tomato juice.

Restrict your diet to these basic foods, then stick with it for two weeks to establish a baseline. Keep a food diary throughout the entire elimination diet process, noting exactly what you eat and when, how you feel, if and when you get a migraine, and anything else that seems important. Don't be surprised if you actually get more headaches during the first few days as your body clears toxic chemicals from its system. But if, after a week or two on the elimination diet, your headaches seem to diminish or even disappear altogether, food triggers or toxins in your system are probably at least part of your problem.

Stick with your hypoallergenic diet during the third week, but pick one food from the trigger list (see the sections on alcohol, amines, caffeine, and food additives earlier in the chapter for complete lists) and gradually add *small* portions of that food, noting any reactions. You may want to try the food you like the most or eat most often, since these foods are quite often trigger foods. Begin by adding one teaspoon of the food to one meal. Take your pulse before eating. Ten minutes after consuming the food, take your pulse again. Does it seem rapid, erratic, or otherwise different from before? Take your pulse again ten minutes later, looking for changes. Also make a note of how you feel. Any obvious changes should be noted in your food diary: nausea, headache, rapid heartbeat, sweating, and so forth. If you feel no reaction, consume the same amount of the food at each meal that day, and see how you do.

The following day, if the food caused no unpleasant reactions, try one tablespoon with each meal. Increase the amount on subsequent days by one tablespoon until you are consuming an entire serving. If you still feel or see no reaction after seven days of testing, the food is probably "safe" and you can resume eating it on a normal basis. Each suspected food should be tested in this way until you can pinpoint your trigger foods. Remember that some foods or additives will only affect you in certain combinations or in certain amounts.

Discovering your trigger foods via the elimination diet is a tricky process and requires a good amount of work—and guesswork—but it can be worth it in the end.

Sample Food Diary

Photocopy this chart—make several copies so you can keep track of your consumption and reactions for several months.

Day	Time	Kind & amount of food consumed	Pulse before eating	Pulse 10 minutes after eating	Pulse 20 minutes after eating	Reactions

Chapter 7

—◀◉▶—

Eliminating Environmental and Other Triggers

- Do you live in a humid environment?
- Do you smoke or share your living or working space with a smoker?
- Is your workplace lit by fluorescent lights?
- Do you spend a lot of time sitting at a desk or working on a computer?
- Do you sleep with feather pillows and a down comforter?
- Do you live with pets?
- Have you recarpeted, repainted, or refurnished your house within the last six months?
- Do you live in an area with high pollen counts?
- Do you wear perfume or use perfumed products (including household cleaners)?
- Does the air filter on your heater go unchanged (or uncleaned) for longer than a month at a time?
- Do you have a gas heater, gas range, or wood-burning fireplace in your home?
- Do you have drapes, carpeting, and upholstered furniture in your home?

If you answered yes to any of these questions, your migraines may be triggered by your environment. Just as certain foods, their components and/or additives can bring on hypersensitive reactions that trigger your migraines, so can the chemicals, particles, plants, animals, noise, light, heat, and other things that are a part of our everyday environment. Dust mites, yeasts, molds, algae, smoke, carbon monoxide, flickering lights, and toxic chemicals are just a few of the things that can trigger migraines in sensitive individuals. Although it will take plenty of time and effort, it can be well worth your while to purify your environment as much as possible and keep it that way. Then, at worst, you've created a healthier environment for yourself and your family. And at best, your migraines may ease up—or even disappear entirely.

HOW ALLERGIES TRIGGER MIGRAINES

Certain substances in the environment—for example, the mold that forms at the base of that dripping faucet in your bathroom—pose absolutely no problem for the average person. But if you should happen to be one of the lucky ones whose systems are hypersensitive to that mold (or, more correctly, the spores that the mold releases into the air), your immune system will go on the rampage. That's because for you mold is an allergen, which means that it triggers an allergic reaction that can leave you with a stuffy nose, itchy, watering eyes, bronchial congestion, headaches, hives, or a skin rash. While the average person wouldn't be affected by the presence of mold spores, your immune system mistakenly identifies them as real threats to the health and integrity of your body. Alarmed, it calls out the troops, sending legions of antibodies called immunoglobulin E, or IgE, into battle.

A specific kind of IgE antibody can be manufactured for almost every kind of allergen the body encounters (including the mold spores). As these IgE antibodies are produced, they make their way to the surface of the *mast cells,* the cells that trigger allergy symptoms. There they hang on for dear life. These mast cells are found in all the tissues in your body, but especially in those that come in contact with the environment, such as the mucous membrane linings in the nose, throat, lungs, reproductive organs, and intestinal tract. The mast cells contain a high-powered inflammatory agent known as *histamine.* When a certain amount of IgE antibodies have been produced and have taken their places on the mast cells, these cells become primed and ready, like loaded guns with a finger on the trigger. Then, the next time you inhale another mold spore, and another IgE antibody moves into position, the mast cells will open the floodgates, releasing the histamine and triggering an inflammation response, better known as an allergic reaction.

How does this bring on your headaches? As a part of the inflammation process, the blood vessels (including those in your head and face) become more porous, allowing the blood's fluid and cells to seep into nearby tissues. The irritated blood vessels widen as tissues become even more inflamed. Does this sound familiar? It should, because it's a major part of the migraine process. Although true allergy headaches are relatively rare, many environmental factors *do* have the potential to assault the nervous system and trigger a full-on migraine attack. That's why it may be worth your while to reduce or eliminate as many of these factors as possible. Ask yourself these questions:

- Are you exposed to the chemical solvents found in nail polish remover, window-cleaning fluids, and other common beauty, household cleaning, and repair items?

- Do you use makeup, lotions, bath items, and other cosmetics?
- Can your pets be getting your dander up?
- Do you have drapes, carpets, upholstered furniture, voluminous bedding, or other places where large amounts of dust can "hide"?
- Do your pillows contain feathers or down?
- Do you have dripping taps, damp basements, or other areas in your house where moisture collects?
- Do you have pollinating plants in your house? Are your windows wide open when the pollen count is high?
- Are you exposed to cigarette or other kinds of smoke?

A yes answer to any of these questions tells you where to begin cleansing your home environment.

HOUSEHOLD HUMIDITY

One of the best ways to kill a couple of birds with one stone is to reduce the humidity in your home, since high humidity makes for a friendly breeding ground for mold, yeast, algae, and dust mites. You can do a lot to reduce humidity in your home by taking simple measures like fixing dripping taps, or buying and using a room dehumidifier. Or, if humidity is a real problem, you may have to try more complicated solutions, such as installing a vapor barrier and insulating your basement ceiling. Consider the tips listed opposite, from the simplest to the most complex measures, and take into account the climate in which you live. (Those who live in the rain forest of Washington State may need to follow these suggestions more carefully than those who live in the high desert of Arizona!)

- Keep your house well ventilated by opening windows and doors whenever possible.
- Air out steamy bathrooms immediately after use, and towel off shower walls, shower doors, bathtubs, counters, and mirrors.
- Wipe condensation off of windows, windowsills, glass doors, and fish tanks regularly.
- Stay away from greenhouses, compost heaps, basements, cellars, and other damp areas where mold is likely to grow.
- Get rid of your waterbed.
- Watch for signs of black or green mold growth in damp areas, and scrub it off with diluted chlorine bleach or cleanser.
- Wash your shower curtain in hot water and chlorine bleach.
- Clean out the refrigerator and garbage containers often to keep mold from growing.
- Use a dehumidifier, especially in the bathroom, laundry room, kitchen, and bedroom to keep humidity between 40 and 50 percent.
- Fix faucets that drip.
- Get your heating and air-conditioning system cleaned and checked. (Mold spores are easily circulated via the air vents in your house.)
- Use paint that has a paint-mold inhibitor added.
- Remove the carpet from the bathroom floor.
- Install gutters and downspouts to take rainwater away from the house so it won't seep into the foundation or basement.
- Install and use exhaust fans in the bathroom and kitchen to help remove humidity.
- Add insulation to the basement ceiling and install a vapor barrier.

DISMISS THE DUST!

Dust mites are tiny, microscopic animals that live in soft furnishings like carpets, bedding, pillows, upholstered furniture, and drapes, and feed on dust and skin scales. Actually, the dust mite itself isn't really the problem; it's the animal's droppings that are the true allergen. Light as dust, the droppings fly through the air and into our respiratory systems, where they can set off symptoms similar to hay fever—or perhaps a migraine attack.

A favorite hangout of the dust mite is your bed. Not only do they love to burrow into those dust-catching mattresses, pillows, and fabrics, they crave the warmth and humidity created by the combination of perspiration and plenty of insulation. Unfortunately, you probably spend more time in your bed, with your nose pressed firmly into your pillow, than you do anywhere else. So as you begin your war on dust and dust mites, look first to your bedroom and particularly your bed:

- Wash your bedding weekly in the hottest water (130 degrees Fahrenheit); you may want to add a special laundry additive that kills dust mites.
- Avoid the use of down-filled blankets or feather pillows (dust mites love them!); use hypoallergenic ones instead, but stay away from foam rubber.
- Put special microporous ("dust mite–proof") covers on pillows, mattresses, and box springs.
- Consider purchasing pillows made with dust mite–proof barriers.
- Replace your pillows yearly, the mattresses every few years.
- Vacuum at least once a week (more often if necessary) and don't forget to vacuum under the bed.
- Don't use the under-bed area to store things. Those odds and

ends trap dust and make it less likely that you'll vacuum "down under."

- Get rid of stuffed animals, if you can bear to part with them. If not, put them in plastic bags, seal them tight, and place them in the freezer overnight to kill dust mites. Then wash them to get rid of dust. Repeat this "cold cleaning" process every month or so.

It's particularly important that you pay attention to forced-air heating systems, which can circulate a great deal of dust:

- Have your heating system cleaned and checked. Install filters over the heating vents in each room and be sure to clean them once a month.
- Or, if your heating system comes equipped with air filters that are changeable, consider getting an electrostatic filter. These are very effective at trapping dust, mold, pollen, and other irritants, but they *must* be cleaned once a month if they're to remain effective.
- You might also consider using an electric radiator in place of forced-air heating.

In general:

- Get a vacuum with a microfilter, or use microfiltration vacuum bags. Otherwise, you may be spewing a good deal of dust back into the environment as you vacuum.
- Change vacuum bags often. A full bag can release even more dust than it accumulates.
- Clean your carpets often with a tannic acid solution to kill dust mites.
- Wash your curtains or drapes frequently in very hot water. If you really have a problem with dust, you might consider get-

ting rid of your drapes *and* your carpets in favor of shades and hardwood floors.
• Stay away from blinds, as they trap dust.

WHAT ABOUT PETS?

It's entirely possible that your headaches are related to sensitivity to animal dander. Dander is a combination of fur, skin scales, and protein that, in some people, can set off an allergic reaction almost instantaneously. The most allergenic animals are cats, who continually groom themselves by licking their coats to remove dirt and loose hair. That may make them seem like the cleanest animals in the world, but when their saliva dries, it emits a protein that floats through the air and is extremely allergenic to many people. The protein can continue to float (and cause allergic reactions) long after the cat has left the scene permanently: for weeks, months, or even years!

Cats may be the most allergenic of animals, but birds, dogs, hamsters, mice, and just about anything else that has fur or feathers can also touch off reactions. If you've got pets, take this simple test to help determine whether or not they're contributing to your headaches. Leave them at a friend's house for a week or two and see if your headaches ease up. If they do, you may want to make your house a pet-free zone. You may also want to visit an allergist for a more definitive diagnosis. If you are, in fact, allergic to your pets, it might be a good idea to leave them with your friend permanently. But if you want to continue to live with pets in spite of your allergies, consider these tips:

• Keep your pets outside as much as possible.
• If you must have them inside, keep them confined to one

room (preferably a room where you *don't* spend the bulk of your time).

- Don't allow them to get on the furniture.
- Keep pets out of your bedroom—and, particularly, out of your bed.
- Wash your hands after touching your pets.
- Have them bathed by a professional groomer.
- Any brushing or grooming that's done at home should be done outside, by someone other than yourself!

INDOOR AIR POLLUTION

You probably think that environmental pollution is something that lurks outside your door—but the air indoors can actually be even more polluted! We live in a virtual chemical soup, and, to make matters worse, our homes are so well insulated that these chemicals tend to hang in the air indefinitely. For some people, even one whiff of cigarette smoke, perfume, cleaning solution, or some other pungent odor is enough to set a migraine into motion. Just imagine what constant exposure to such odors must produce! Do your best to reduce or eliminate the odors of gas stove emissions, chemical solvents, clothes that have been dry cleaned, household cleansers, perfume, cosmetics, fabric treatments, hairspray, air fresheners, and any other chemical smells that assault the nervous system. Then, become a fresh air fanatic. Weather permitting, keep your house as well ventilated as possible. Open the windows and install screen doors so you can let in plenty of fresh air (unless it's pollen season and that's a problem for you). Your air conditioner can help filter the air during hot weather. Just make sure it's well maintained and the vents are clean.

Secondly, consider buying an air-filtration system. The best ones are the HEPA ("high-efficiency particulate air") filters, which can trap 99.97 percent of all airborne particles that are 0.3 microns or larger. That means dust, dust mite droppings, animal dander, mold, pollen, viruses, and bacteria will be siphoned out and trapped in the filter, instead of continuing to circulate through the air you breathe. You'll need to clean or change the filter every couple of months, but you may be able to spare yourself some migraine episodes just by investing in one (or more) of these little machines. They're widely available just about anywhere that kitchen appliances are sold, and many cost less than $100. I suggest you put one in your bedroom, one in the room where you spend the most time (such as the family room), and one in the room where your pets (if any) spend time.

Finally, consider these general tips for reducing toxins in your environment:

- Replace harsh household cleansers with environmentally friendly ones. Scrubbing chores can be done with a mixture of baking soda and water, and windows will sparkle when cleansed with a quart of water to which a quarter cup of vinegar has been added. Lavender essential oil (available from aromatherapists) plus rubbing alcohol makes a good disinfectant.
- Avoid aerosol spray products.
- Always opt for the unscented rather than the scented product.
- Use hypoallergenic soaps and cosmetics.
- If you must use hairspray, use the pump-spray variety and apply it next to an open window.
- Avoid perfume and perfumed products.
- Wear natural fabrics and stay away from those that require dry cleaning.

- Stop smoking and ban smoking in your home or in your presence.
- Don't use wood-burning stoves or fireplaces (too smoky).
- The chemical finishes put on new carpets, drapes, or upholstered furniture will release toxins into the air for up to two months in a process called *outgassing.* Use your HEPA air filter and keep doors and windows open as much as possible during this time.
- After painting with oil-based paints, installing carpeting, draperies, or fabric furniture (such as couches, chairs), or refinishing wood floors, make sure the house is well ventilated for at least eight weeks. A HEPA filter with a special odor-absorbing (charcoal) insert can help a lot.
- Home improvement projects that require the use of polyurethane varnish, spray paint, soldering, or formaldehyde-containing substances should be done outside, away from the house if possible. Dry the items completely and let vapors subside before introducing them into the home environment.

OUTDOOR TOXINS

Smog, especially car exhaust, can be a major source of migraine trouble, producing chemicals like nitrogen dioxide, ground-level ozone, benzene, and carbon monoxide. Sulfur dioxide, a by-product of emissions from power plants, constricts the airways and may contribute to lower levels of blood oxygen, triggering headaches. Pesticides, natural gas, and other noxious inhalants or chemicals emanating from farms, factories, or construction sites can assault your nervous and respiratory systems, resulting in migraines. And even something as natural as ragweed pollen or the molds that form on decomposing wood or leaves may cause a war to break out inside your skull.

If your headaches seem to get worse when you spend time outdoors, try to discern whether or not your symptoms create a pattern. Are they worse during the spring and fall, when the pollen is out in full force? Do smoggy days affect you more than clear days? How about wind? Once you figure out which seasons or kinds of weather are the worst for you, try the following during your "headache" times:

Indoors and Around the House

- Keep windows and doors closed.
- Especially during heavy pollution or high pollen days, use an air filter or air conditioner to keep your indoor air as clean and particulate-free as possible.
- Hire someone to do the heavy chemical work, like painting your house or applying fertilizers and/or pesticides.

Outdoors

- If you have to go outdoors during periods of heavy pollution or pollen, wear a filter mask (available at hardware stores). Then shower, wash your hair, and wash your clothes once you get home.
- Avoid walking in the woods or other moist places, especially during the fall, if you're sensitive to mold.
- If you jog around the neighborhood or otherwise exercise outdoors, do so in the evening, when pollution and pollen counts are lowest.
- When exercising or playing outdoors, stay away from heavy traffic and highly industrialized areas. In other words, don't

jog or bike down heavily trafficked boulevards. Look for a relatively car-free area instead.

While Driving

- Keep your car windows closed when driving.
- Use the air conditioner as a built-in filter. (Set the system to recycle the air in your car rather than draw air in from outside.)

HOW'S THE WEATHER?

If you've got migraines, the weather can be much more than just a safe topic for elevator conversation. Certain types of weather—springtime weather in general, the hot, humid days of summer, and the sudden onset of storm fronts—can increase both the frequency and severity of migraines. Springtime encourages migraines because of the sudden proliferation of allergens in the air. The heat and humidity of summer encourage mold growth, the release of grass pollens, and the proliferation of heavy smog. But sudden rainstorms may be the most notorious weather-related cause of migraines.

How can a rainstorm instigate a migraine? Many migraine sufferers seem to be extremely sensitive to changes in barometric pressure. Some people, in fact, know in advance that a storm is coming because they can feel a migraine building. The sudden increase in humidity caused by a storm also fosters an automatic increase in allergens (molds, spores, dust mites, etc.), which may trigger migraines.

Changes in the concentration of ions in the air may also be the culprit. Ions are atoms that have either too many or too few electrons, making them either positively or negatively charged. As the weather changes, so does the ratio of positive to negative ions. In general, storms increase the proliferation of positive ions, which like to float freely through the air. Brewing storms also spur the release of extra amounts of pollen grains and spores, making the air even more laden with allergens. But negative ions like to stick to surfaces and cling to the positively charged particles in the air. Negative ions are better for your health, since they attach themselves to airborne allergens, then stick to surfaces like doors or counters, instead of floating into your respiratory system. Ionizer units are designed to "inhale" positive ions through a filter, then give them a negative charge before releasing them into the air. They may be of help, especially when positive ion ratios are high.

What can you do about migraines caused by the weather? Not a lot, unfortunately, other than staying inside during humid weather and periods when storms are brewing, using an ionizer, and following the suggestions outlined above for handling outdoor toxins. Investing in a good home dehumidifier may also help. If humidity and weather changes are severe problems for you, you may want to consider moving to another climate. For most people, though, it's enough just to exercise a little caution. You can also help yourself if you improve your resistance to headaches with other approaches such as regular aerobic exercise, biofeedback, and the triple therapy.

MIGRAINES IN THE WORKPLACE

Is your job giving you a headache (and not just because it's a pain in the neck)? Actually, jobs and workplaces can be important contributing factors to migraines. Air-conditioning systems that recirculate toxic, chemical-laden air, noxious chemicals used on the job, secondhand smoke, fumes from plastic and/or fabric furnishings, and the regular fumigation of office buildings can bring on migraines or make them worse. Bright or flashing lights, computer screens, flickering fluorescent lights, poor lighting, too much reading or close work can cause migraines related to eyestrain. Temperatures that are too high or low may contribute to headaches. And poor posture (often due to "ergonomically incorrect" workstations) can exacerbate migraines by putting undue pressure on the nerves that serve the head, face, and neck. Finally, noisy environments can assault the nervous system and either cause migraines or make them worse. To make your workplace as migraine-free as possible, consider the following:

- Identify the headache triggers in your area, and take a poll of your fellow office workers to see if they're having problems, too. If so, you'll have more ammunition when you ask for changes to be made.
- Check with management or your company's human resources department to see what they are willing to do to correct workplace conditions. The National Organization of Legal Advocates for the Environmentally Injured (phone number 404-264-4445) can advise you of your legal rights as an employee. If you're a member of a union, they should also be able to help.
- Bring green plants to work to help clean the air. Certain plants have a proven ability to clear various toxins from the air. Spider ferns, Boston ferns, chrysanthemums, and English ivy, for example, can clean up such airborne toxins as benzene, trichlorethylene, formaldehyde, and acetone. Aloe vera, ficus, philodendron, and poinsettias are also effective. Figure three eight-inch potted plants for each 100 square feet of office space.

- Lighting should be sufficient but not glaring. To minimize strain, use a desk lamp or overhead fixture that provides soft incandescent light that is adequate to the task. Don't overdo it or underdo it.
- Fluorescent lights are known for flickering, even if you can't tell by looking. Use incandescent bulbs instead. If you can't replace fluorescent lights in the office, you may want to turn off the overhead fluorescents and use a table lamp with an incandescent bulb instead.
- See your eye doctor to determine if your glasses or contacts need adjustment.
- Use a glare guard on your computer screen or turn down the contrast to avoid assaulting your eyes.
- Always close the cover on the copy machine before making copies. (That bright flash of light may trigger a migraine.) Also, wear sunglasses whenever you go outdoors to reduce the glare of bright sunlight.
- Take breaks from the computer every half hour or so. Get up, stretch, walk around, and rest your eyes.

If your workplace is causing too many problems that can't be adjusted or fixed, think about finding another job.

SIT UP AND TAKE NOTICE!

Our bodies were never designed to sit as much as nearly all of us do. Think about it: You sit in your car to drive to work; you arrive and (most likely) spend the morning sitting at a desk or in front of a computer; you drive to a restaurant for lunch where you sit down to take your meal; you drive back to work; spend the rest of the day sitting at your desk, then sit in your car to drive home. Once you're home, you sit and read the paper, sit to eat dinner, sit with the kids to do homework, and sit in front of the television before going to bed.

People from primitive cultures rarely sit. Instead, they stand, squat, or lie down on the hard ground. Because of this, their backs and necks tend to stay in proper alignment, balanced over the pelvis. But we in the modern world hunch over our desk work, crane our necks to see our computer screens, and constantly angle our heads down—an unnatural position. The result: chronically tense back and neck muscles, which can put painful pressure on the nerves servicing the head and face, initiating migraine headaches. (Those who hold the phone receiver by scrunching their shoulder to their ear with the receiver in between are just asking for head and neck trouble!) Because we spend so much time sitting, it's important that we learn to do so correctly. The science of using the body in the least stressful ways is called *ergonomics,* and experts in that field have come up with the following suggestions for minimizing the stress and pain associated with working at a desk:

- Sit up straight in your chair, with your head centered above your shoulders—not pushed forward or pulled back.
- Shoulders should be relaxed and pulled back to your body's midline, just like they are when you're standing with good posture.
- Your computer screen should be placed so that your eyes focus either straight ahead or just below.
- Your chair should have a firm seat back with a curve that matches the curve in your lower back. Sit with your buttocks pushed all the way to the back of the seat and your back resting against the seat back. (Sitting on the edge of your seat, leaning forward as you work, stresses your back. So does slouching back into your chair with buttocks sliding forward and chair back supporting your upper back only.)

- The chair seat should angle slightly so that your knees are slightly higher than your hips. Otherwise, your lower back will want to come away from the backrest and muscle tension will increase.
- Chair height should be set so that your feet rest flat on the floor. If that's not possible, put a footrest or books under your feet to achieve the proper angle.
- The arms of your chair should be adjustable and positioned so that your forearms, wrists, and hands are in a straight line as you type, forming a 90-degree angle to your body.
- Your keyboard should be level with your elbows.
- Take frequent breaks—look away from your computer screen or other close work, stretch, get up, and walk around. Your body will thank you for it, and you'll be more efficient in the long run.

MOTION

Another common migraine trigger is motion, which commonly manifests itself as car sickness, seasickness, or air sickness and can segue into a miserable headache. No one knows why motion can bring on migraines, but those who are prone to motion sickness seem to be somewhat more likely to develop migraines than the average person. If motion happens to be one of your triggers, do what you can to avoid long trips, get plenty of fresh air whenever possible, sit in the front seat of the car, and make several stops along the way to regain your bearings.

HIGH ALTITUDE AND CARBON MONOXIDE

High altitude and carbon monoxide have one thing in common: They both deprive the brain of much-needed oxygen. Everyone knows that the air is thin up there in mountainous areas, and that it takes a few days to get adjusted to the lower levels of oxygen. Carbon monoxide has the same effect, but for a different reason. The highly unstable carbon monoxide molecules latch on to hemoglobin, a protein-iron compound in the blood that carries oxygen to the cells and carbon dioxide away from them. Because carbon monoxide takes up the same "seats" on the hemoglobin that oxygen should be using, less and less oxygen is transported to the cells.

A lack of oxygen (for whatever reason) causes the blood vessels in the brain to relax and widen so that more blood (and therefore more oxygen) can make its way to the brain cells. And that means a greater propensity toward migraines.

To avoid carbon monoxide–induced migraines, do the following:

- Make sure gas-powered cooking ranges, fuel-burning heaters, furnaces, and chimneys are inspected regularly to ensure proper function and no leakage of carbon monoxide.
- Consider replacing your gas range with an electric one.
- Install a carbon monoxide detector in your home.
- Don't run your car in a closed garage.
- Ban cigarette smoking in your home and in your presence. (Carbon monoxide is a by-product of cigarette smoke.)

To prevent or ease migraines due to high altitudes:

- Exercise prior to traveling to higher altitudes in order to improve the conditioning of your body.

- Try supplemental vitamin C (1000 mg a day) to help ease the effects of high altitudes.
- Inhale pure oxygen (available in tanks at medical supply stores).
- Wait it out. Within about three days, your body will automatically make greater amounts of hemoglobin to compensate for the lower levels of available oxygen.
- Sometimes a doctor can prescribe a drug called Diamox (acetazolamide), a unique diuretic that has to be taken for a day or two prior to ascent.

All the things suggested in this chapter seem like a lot of work. But if making some changes can reduce or eliminate your migraines, it's worth the effort.

Chapter 8

—◄○►—

Taking the Edge Off

Since stress is a major trigger of migraines, it makes sense that reducing the stress in your life can help lessen the number of headaches you get. There's been a great deal written on ways to reduce stress, most of which boils down to two ideas: Close the door on potential stress, and crowd out current stress by thinking happy and fun thoughts.

To close the door on potential stress, you've got to prevent stress from getting into your head in the first place. How do you do that? Begin by reminding yourself that most of the time stress is just a matter of opinion. Yes, there are some situations that are absolutely and unavoidably stressful. For example, being on the front line during a battle is extremely stressful because of the very real possibility of injury or death. Experiencing a death in the family or going through a divorce is highly stressful because these involve major life changes. But most things are "optional stress." You *choose* to respond to the fact that you're late and caught in traffic by cursing the other drivers and pounding your fists on the steering wheel. You could just as easily choose to accept the fact that you're going to be late, and perhaps pull over, make a call and let the person you're supposed to meet know when you'll be there.

Now, suppose your plumber did a poor job repairing your pipes and has refused to give you a refund. You can scream and holler, which will push your stress levels and your blood pressure sky-high. You can then spend the next two years telling everyone who will listen about how that plumber cheated you, which will continue to make your stress levels and blood pressure rise. Or you can sit down and calmly write a letter detailing the problem, send it to the proper regulatory agencies, and then *forget about it.*

Similarly, you can go to the movies and stew about the jerk in the row in back of you who insists on talking and rattling candy wrappers throughout the duration of the show. You can shoot dirty looks at him, hiss at him to be quiet, and, as a result, find yourself completely unable to concentrate. Or you can get up and find another seat where you can relax and get into the movie.

We're all subjected to unpleasant people and situations every day. We can relish the chance to get angry and stressed out, or we can close the doors on stress by refusing to get angry, declining to go over infuriating situations again and again in our minds or conversations, and simply forgetting about it.

Of course, it's unrealistic to expect that we'll never get upset. Sometimes we get rip-roaring mad, or realize that a lot of little stresses have built up inside. That's when we have to push negative thoughts out of our heads. There are lots of simple ways to do that. For example, you can:

- *Do something completely different.* Break away from your routine every once in a while. If you always go to the movies on the weekend, try taking a drive out to the desert or mountains instead. If you always vacation at the beach, try something new, like exploring a city you've never visited before. If you usually spend your evenings reading a novel or watching television, go bowling one night a week or join a club. Occasionally doing something new can add some excitement and fun to your life, give you something to look forward to, and help you break away from the same old thought patterns.

- *Exercise.* Walk, run, lift weights, swim, bicycle, play volleyball, baseball, soccer, or any number of other fun sports. But remember, fun is the key. If you play to win at all costs, if you *have* to be the best on your team or if you *have* to be perfect, you won't have much fun. Instead, you'll be adding to your stress load. I know a middle-aged couple who ballroom dance for pleasure. They're like Fred Astaire and Ginger Rogers, waltzing, fox-trotting, and cha-cha-ing across the floor. They look great, and from the big smiles on their faces you can tell they're also having a great time. "But it wasn't always like that," the husband explains. "We used to try so hard to be perfect we wound up fighting all the time. I'd say her little finger wasn't tilted just so, she'd say my shoulder was angled back. We almost strangled each other several times until we agreed to stop trying to be perfect and just dance. Now we have a great time dancing. And nobody cares if her pinky or my shoulder are right or wrong. It's so much more relaxing."

- *Meditate.* This is a passive way of relieving stress. Just sit and look at nothing. Think about nothing. Do nothing. No noise, no distractions, no demands, no schedules, no projects, no kids. Just peace, quiet, and an empty mind. Well, not entirely empty. It's hard to turn the thinking off, to prevent thoughts from intruding on your mental silence. Meditation is about learning to ignore those stray thoughts, letting them slide quietly off your mental blackboard and into oblivion. As little as twenty minutes of meditation a day, several days a week, can help reduce your stress level. Meditation classes are often taught at yoga studios, gyms, as extension classes at community colleges, or by private trainers. Sometimes larger businesses offer courses in meditation to their employees. Or you may learn the techniques through a book. Any way you learn to do it, meditation is an excellent way to relieve stress and keep things in perspective.

- *Have fun!*—Try to have a little fun every day. Start the day by reading the comic section in the newspaper, or get into one of those joke-swapping circles on the Internet. Don't work through lunch, and take regular breaks at work. See your friends often (but don't get into gripe sessions). Read novels that are fun, interesting, and give you a chance to escape for a while. Try singing; you'd be surprised how much fun that can be. Sing in church, sing along with a CD, get together with some friends for a singalong in someone's living room, or join a choir. How about getting involved in a hobby or doing arts and crafts? Or taking a completely casual, no-stress night out with the girls—or the boys?

- *Make a list, check it twice, and toss it out.* I have a friend who runs a bustling public relations firm. He tells me that he has more paperwork than he can handle, so he puts each piece of paper into one of five piles on his desk. The piles are labeled: "Do Immediately," "Do Very Soon," "Get More Info," "Delegate," and "Can Wait." He told me, "Every once in a while I go through the 'Can Wait' pile and I throw out half the papers. Either I never needed to deal with them in the first place, or whatever they were about is no longer important. I've seen this happen over and over again through the years.

So many of the things I think are absolutely vital and must be handled right now aren't that important. I don't deal with them, but the world doesn't come to an end. That can only mean they weren't really that important to begin with. I only thought they were."

Is everything on your mental to-do list absolutely, irrevocably crucial? Or are you, like most of us, making minor things more important than they need to be and allowing them to stress you? Perhaps you should try to make a list of all the things you have to do and arrange them in order of importance. Then tear off the items at the end and toss them out. There's a good chance you'll never miss them—but you *will* notice that you're not as harried and rushed as usual.

- *Learn to recognize and control body reactions.* One fifty-one-year-old woman I know named Nina is able to sense her migraines coming on, even before the aura strikes. "As soon as I feel the first little twinge of an oncoming migraine, I sit down in a quiet room, close my eyes, and envision the blood vessels in my head staying at normal size. I silently tell myself that they're not getting wider or narrower, and I mentally see them staying at normal size. I silently tell myself that my brain chemistry will remain stable, my blood pressure will remain normal, my fingers will stay warm, and my stomach will stay peaceful. A lot of times that does the trick. I don't get the headache."

Nina learned this technique in biofeedback, a therapy that teaches you how to recognize and control some important body functions. During a typical biofeedback session, you'll be hooked up to an instrument that monitors your temperature or the electrical activity of certain muscles. But the instruments do more than register changes in your body: They show you what's happening. You can "see" your muscle tension as a line that moves across the screen; you can "hear" the electrical activity of your muscles as a tone gets louder or softer, or perhaps higher or lower in pitch. As you "look at" and "listen to" what's happening in your body, you practice relaxation techniques. And you can see how the relaxation actually changes your body as your heartbeat slows, your muscles relax, and so on.

When you become proficient at this, you, like Nina, can slip into your relaxation mode and help control certain body responses without being hooked up to the biofeedback machines. More importantly, you may learn to do relaxation exercises on the go, while talking to someone, walking, or doing anything else. During these biofeedback mini-sessions you'll subconsciously and effortlessly monitor your muscle tension. This will help you head off the stressful situations that may trigger your migraines. It will also help you deal with the stress that comes from your headaches.

Many of my patients tell me that once they find a way to reduce the stress in their lives, a good portion of their headaches seem to melt away, as well. The stress relievers listed above are just a few of many, many others, including massage, qi gong, hot baths, and so forth. It really doesn't matter what you do as long as it works for you. Try them all—at the very least you'll have a pleasant, relaxing time.

Chapter 9

◀◉▶

Walking It Off

- Do you consider the TV remote control to be the greatest invention since penicillin?
- Do you drive around the parking lot looking for the closest parking space to the door, even if there are plenty of available spaces farther away?
- Do you drive just about everywhere you go, even if you're only going several blocks?
- Has it been years since you've exercised regularly?
- Are sports or physically active games something you left behind with your teenage years?
- Do you think of exercise as work?
- Do you shun exercise because you just don't have the time?
- Do you think you have to put in at least thirty straight minutes of huffing and puffing per session for exercise to be of any benefit?

- Do stress and tension play a part in your migraines?
- Do you find it hard to relax, even when you've got the time?

If you answered yes more than a couple of times, a lack of exercise may be playing a role in your migraine headaches.

When you've got a migraine, there's no question: The last thing you want to do is go for a jog in the park. And I wouldn't suggest that you do, although I have had patients who managed to "exercise away" a migraine in its early stages. What I *do* suggest is that you incorporate regular exercise into your life as a way to prevent migraines. Frequent exercise, with its many beneficial effects on overall health, has also been shown to boost the threshold of headache pain—that is, regular exercise makes it less likely that you'll feel the effects of a headache. And that translates to fewer and milder migraines.

WHAT EXERCISE CAN DO
TO HELP COMBAT MIGRAINES

Exercise can help fight migraines in myriad ways, both internal and external. Some of the migraine-busting effects of regular workouts include:

- *Lowered stress levels and increased relaxation.* Stress causes negative changes in the body, including blood vessel constriction, muscle tension, and the release of stress chemicals into the bloodstream, all of which can increase the potential for migraines. Relaxation, on the other hand, is the antithesis of stress, widening the blood vessels, decreasing muscle tension, and eating up those excess stress chemicals.
- *Increased circulation of both blood and lymph.* The net effect is that more oxygen is brought to the tissues, while toxins are

cleared away faster. Lack of oxygen and toxic buildup are two potent instigators of migraines.

- *Increased production of endorphins.* There is some evidence that migraine sufferers may produce lower amounts of endorphins, the body's natural painkiller, than those who don't get migraines. Also, the frequent use of pain relievers (a common practice with migraineurs) can actually reduce endorphin production, leading to an increased propensity to feel pain. Exercise can help counteract both of these conditions.
- *Reduced fatigue.* Those who exercise regularly tend to have higher overall energy levels and a greater resistance to fatigue, one of the common triggers of migraines.
- *Improved sleep quality and duration.* When the body undergoes physical stress (as it does during exercise), it counterbalances that stress by inducing greater amounts of deep sleep. Also, the rise and fall of body temperature seen during and after an exercise session may help bring on sleep (if the session occurs three to six hours before bedtime).
- *Improved digestion.* Exercise helps tone abdominal muscles and improves peristalsis, the squeezing action of the digestion system. As a result, transit time through the intestines decreases and waste products are removed from the body more quickly. This lessens the likelihood of constipation and decreases the level of circulating toxins.
- *Reduced incidence of depression and anxiety.* Sensitivity to pain increases with depression and anxiety, but exercise helps counteract that by stimulating endorphin production.

If you could invent a pill that reduced stress, decreased depression and anxiety, improved sleep, and reduced pain, you'd make enough money to send your kids to college *and* take early retirement—on your own private island! But the world doesn't need such a pill. These wonderful "side effects" are free to all those who will get moving!

And you don't have to exhaust yourself in the effort. In the past, scientists believed that the only way to get these benefits was to engage in *aerobic exercise,* like jogging, jumping rope, cycling, or fast dancing—anything that increases your heart rate and your consumption of oxygen. But newer evidence shows that most, if not all, of the pluses can be yours even if you do milder, gentler exercises, like gardening, taking the stairs instead of riding the elevator, or walking at a moderate pace. In 1996, a new program of "kinder, gentler" exercise was recommended by the surgeon general, involving thirty minutes of moderately intensive physical activity just about every day. (Taking off a day or two a week is okay; just space them so that you don't take two days in succession.)

And remember: Engaging in strenuous exercise while you're experiencing a headache can intensify pain and other symptoms. If you feel you must exercise during the course of a headache, do something gentle like easy walking or stretching. If the pain gets worse, stop exercising immediately and retire to a dark, quiet room.

Caution: It is vital that you consult with your physician before beginning, expanding, or changing your exercise program. This is especially true if you are over the age of forty, have any injuries, or suffer from heart disease or other ailments.

TAKE IT IN SMALL BITES

Let's say you like the idea of exercise but you can't seem to find the time, or you really hate the boredom of long workouts. Then you should consider grabbing little "mini" exercise sessions throughout the day. Studies have shown that what matters most is not the length of your exercise session but how much *cumulative* time you spend exercising in a day. In other words, the benefits you get from a thirty-minute brisk walk are not appreciably greater than those you get from a ten-minute bike ride in the morning, a ten-minute jog on the treadmill in the afternoon, and a brisk ten-minute walk in the evening. And, remember, the standard "exercising" activities (walking, jogging, cycling, swimming, etc.) aren't the only kinds of movement that count. Anything that gets you out of your chair for at least ten minutes will be of value, including:

- cleaning out cupboards
- golf
- easy cycling
- house painting
- mopping the floor
- mowing the lawn with a push mower
- Ping-Pong
- playing outdoors with your kids
- pushing a child in a stroller
- raking leaves
- shopping
- sweeping
- swimming
- taking the stairs instead of the elevator
- wallpapering
- washing the car
- washing windows

Remember, your goal should be to work in thirty minutes of exercise every day. Naturally, there will be occasional days when you can't exercise (such as when you've got a migraine or are otherwise ill, when you're injured, etc.), but you'll find it easier to accomplish your daily exercise goal if you don't give yourself a choice. Just get up and move!

OR IT MAY BE WORTH IT TO WORK A LITTLE HARDER . . .

Exercise is no different than a lot of other things in life: You get out of it what you put into it. If you do the minimum, you'll get minimum results. But if you do a little more, you'll probably get better results. Those who do their thirty minutes of easy exercise every day probably will have fewer and milder migraines, but those who are willing to work a little harder may be able to build in extra protection. Researchers have found that aerobic exercise—the kind that gets your heart beating faster and makes you breathe harder—done three or four times a week for as little as twenty minutes, plus daily neck and back stretches, can do much to ward off headaches. But that means twenty minutes in one session (not two ten-minute sessions) because an aerobic exercise is, by definition, exercise that can raise your heart rate and keep it there for at least fifteen to twenty minutes consecutively.

Now, I'm not suggesting that you push yourself to the point where your face turns bright red, you're panting, and your heart feels like it's going to burst. You should just push yourself slightly beyond what you'd normally do. To make sure you're exercising within a safe but effective range, consult the chart for target heart rate ranges opposite. Your goal should be to get your heart beating slightly faster than the lower number but slower than the upper number indicated for your approximate age.

ARE YOU IN "THE ZONE"?

To figure out your heart rate, you'll need to know how to take your pulse accurately and you'll need a watch with a second hand.

To take your pulse, hold your left hand in front of you, at about chest level, with the palm side facing up. Place the index and second fingers of your right hand on the tendon that runs lengthwise down the center of your wrist. Now slide those two fingers slightly to the thumb side of the tendon until they settle into the little hollow that's situated there. You should be able to feel your pulse.

About ten minutes into the middle of your workout, take your pulse. Use a stopwatch or a clock with a second hand, and count the pulse beats for fifteen seconds. Then multiply that number by four and you'll have your heart rate per minute. Check the chart below to see if you are within the proper range for your age. If you're too high, take it a bit easier. Too low? Step up the pace a bit.

Target Heart Rates During Aerobic Exercise

Age	Target zone
20	120–150
25	117–146
30	114–142
35	111–138
40	108–135
45	105–131

50	102–127
55	99–123
60	96–120
65	93–116
70	90–113

LOTS TO CHOOSE FROM

While aerobic exercise may take a little extra effort, it has the advantage of being energizing, fun, and wonderfully diverse. Your choices can range from dancing to sports to cross-country skiing. The best idea is to mix them up; don't get stuck in a rut. Do basketball one day, fast walking the next. Try ballroom dancing (it's surprisingly aerobic if done continuously) or a quick game of racquetball. Remember that you don't need to labor at anything for more than about twenty minutes, unless you want to. But you may be surprised at how quickly the time goes! Consider the following forms of aerobic exercise:

- aerobics
- basketball
- cross-country skiing
- cycling (fast or uphill)
- dancing (fast and/or continuous)
- hiking
- racquetball or squash
- rowing
- running (outdoors or on a treadmill)
- stair climbing
- step exercises

- swimming (fast)
- tennis
- walking (fast or uphill)

WARM-UP IS KING

Although you may be tempted to put on your running shoes and take off like a shot, don't do it. Your body needs to go through a transitional period from its sedentary state ("cold" muscles) through the gradual increase of heart rate and breathing until it reaches its active state, with muscles now thoroughly "warmed" by increased blood and oxygen. Exercising at full bore when you're not warmed up is like trying to fight a battle before all the troops have arrived. You run the risk of muscle injury, exhaustion, and a buildup of lactic acid in the muscles that will translate to a lot of extra soreness tomorrow or the next day. Always take the time to warm your muscles thoroughly before getting into heavy exercise. You can do this by walking at a moderate then brisk pace, doing some light jogging on the treadmill, perhaps some jumping jacks or other calisthenics or some easy cycling. When your face begins to feel warm and you've broken a sweat, you're probably ready to step up the pace.

DOES EXERCISE GIVE YOU A HEADACHE?

For some people, exercise can bring on what's known as an *exertional headache*. That's because the blood vessels in the brain dilate to accommodate the increased need for oxygen, and may overdo it, bringing on a headache. Exertional headaches typically occur in those age forty or older who have just started an exercise program, and can be brought on by strenuous exercise like jogging, aerobics, or weightlifting. But they can also occur during or after sex or a coughing spell, as the heart rate increases and blood flow to the head increases. These headaches usually last only about fifteen or twenty minutes, but can be excruciating. Should you get one, retire to a dark room, lie down, and put a cold cloth on your head. You may wish to stick with low-impact activities like walking, biking, swimming, or using the treadmill until your fitness levels increase and your body becomes more efficient at meeting its oxygen needs. Taking two Advils or aspirins an hour before exercise or sex can sometimes prevent these headaches.

Warning: It is vital that you seek immediate medical attention the first time you have an exertion headache, for in rare cases it may be a sign of a ruptured brain aneurysm, an often deadly condition.

THE MOST RELAXING EXERCISES IN THE WORLD

Aerobic exercises are just a part of the equation when it comes to headache prevention. They rev the body up, burn off excess energy, and get all systems moving. But you also need to bring the body down, relax, and ease all systems into the resting mode. Stretching exercises are the perfect vehicle for relaxation, especially after a workout. But the easier stretches (head rolls, neck stretches, etc.) can be done as part of a warm-up, a cool-down, or a complete stretching routine.

If you're new to stretching or would like to develop a stretching routine, I suggest you join a stretching or yoga class, or see a physical therapist or other expert. There are important techniques you'll need to learn in order to stretch safely and effectively and it's hard to learn them just by reading a book. You really need someone to show you these techniques, then supervise you until you've got them down.

Having said that, I must add that there are certain stretches simple enough to outline here that may help prevent migraines. Mostly they involve the head, neck, and shoulders, and some are subtle enough that they can be done just about anytime or anyplace—whenever you need a break from the tensions of the day. When you feel tension building in your neck, shoulders, or upper back, or if you feel the warning signs of an impending migraine, try one or more of these exercises:

Isometric Exercises

Isometric exercises are those in which certain muscles work against resistance without moving a joint. Often the resistance is provided by the body itself. Isometric exercises involving the neck can help reduce headaches by reducing neck muscle spasm. If done 5–10 times a day, with 10–15 seconds of pressure in each direction, they can strengthen the neck muscles and decrease their risk of spasm.

Isometric Exercise #1

- Sit up straight, head erect, eyes straight forward.
- Place your palm against your forehead with the base of the palm at the bridge of your nose.
- Exert a gentle pressure that steadily increases, while using your neck muscles to keep your head from being pushed backward.
- Hold to the count of 10, then relax.
- Repeat 5–10 times throughout the day.

Isometric Exercise #2

- Assume the same beginning position that you did in the last exercise, but this time place your palm on the side of your head, with the base of the palm just above the top of the ear.
- Again, exert a pressure that gradually increases, while using your neck muscles to keep the head from being pushed to the side.
- Hold to the count of 10, then relax.
- Repeat 5–10 times on each side of the head.

Isometric Exercise #3

- This exercise is similar to the two above, except you interlace your fingers and place the hands at the back of the skull.
- Press, gradually increasing the intensity, using the neck muscles to keep the head from being pushed forward.
- Hold to the count of 10, then relax.
- Repeat 5–10 times throughout the day.

Head Roll

This can be done while sitting at your desk, riding on the subway, or waiting at a stoplight. It's good for relieving tension in the neck and upper back.

- Sit up or stand up straight and drop your head all the way forward as if touching your chin to the base of your neck. Hold for 2 counts.
- Roll your head gently toward the left shoulder, as if trying to touch your ear to your shoulder. (Don't scrunch your shoulder toward your ear.) Hold for 2 counts.

- Roll your head toward the back and hold for 2 counts.
- Roll your head toward your right shoulder, and hold it there for 2 counts.
- Roll your head forward to the starting position.
- Repeat this gentle circular rolling of the head, for a total of 4 times to the left, then 4 times to the right.

Neck Stretch

Tension in the neck muscles can help bring on a migraine or make an existing one worse. Try this as soon as you realize that your neck is "knotting up."

- Sit up straight, facing forward, eyes about horizon level. Continue to face forward as you drop your head gently to the right, with your right ear directly over your right shoulder.
- Keeping your head in its "dropped" position, place your right hand over the top of your head and your left hand on top of your left shoulder.
- Gently press down with both hands. You should feel a nice stretch along the left side of your neck. Hold for 4 counts.
- Release the pressure and let your head assume its natural upright position.
- Repeat on the other side, dropping your head to the left to stretch the right side of the neck. Do this at least 3 times per side.

Look Both Ways

Here's another one that can help relieve neck tension and maintain neck range of motion. Just be sure you do it gently!

- Stand or sit up straight, facing forward with eyes at horizon level. Slowly turn your head toward the right as far as you can and hold it there for 4 counts.
- Maintain that position while you place the fingertips of your hand along the jawline of the left side of your face.
- Gently exert enough pressure to turn your head slightly farther to the right. Hold for 4 counts.
- Release the pressure and turn your head back toward the front.
- Repeat on the left side. Do this exercise twice on each side.

Oblique Neck Stretch

In the "Look Both Ways" exercise, you faced forward and then faced the side, theoretically a difference of about 90 degrees. In this exercise, you face only halfway toward the side, about 45 degrees, to stretch the muscles that run through your upper back at an oblique angle.

- Stand or sit up straight, facing forward, eyes at horizon level. Turn your head about 45 degrees to the right (halfway between facing straight forward and facing all the way to the side), while keeping your head level.
- Put your right hand over the top of your head, palm clasping the back of your head.
- Gently pull your head down, attempting to touch the chin to the chest. Hold for 4 counts.
- Release and bring your head slowly back up to the starting position.
- Repeat on the left side. Do this exercise at least 4 times on each side.

Shrugging Shoulders

Many people hold a great deal of tension in their shoulders and at the sides and base of the neck. This exercise will help you learn to extend your neck and press your shoulders toward the ground, relieving tension and improving posture. Think of a ballet dancer's long neck and head held high while you do this one.

• Stand or sit up straight, with head up and eyes at horizon level. Slowly shrug your shoulders and bring them up as high as you can, as if trying to touch them to your ears. Hold for a count of 2.
• Keeping your head level, eyes straight ahead, slowly relax your shoulders and return them to their normal position.
• Press your shoulders down as you lengthen your neck upward. (Think of two little elves, one on top of each of your shoulders, pressing down on them.) Hold for a count of 2.
• Repeat, first shrugging your shoulders, and then pressing them down as you lengthen your neck. Do this exercise slowly, at least 6 times.

Alternating Stretch

This is a good warm-up stretch, one that can get the blood going and help you lift your chest so that the lungs can expand more fully. But you'll have to stand up to do it, so it's probably not a great one for the office!

• Stand up straight, with your legs together, feet pointing straight ahead. Raise both arms above your head, keeping the tops of your shoulders pressed down toward the floor (i.e., don't shrug your shoulders).

- Lift your right arm, stretching it as if to touch the ceiling with your fingers. You should feel a good pull along your right side.
- Then lift your left arm and stretch it toward the ceiling, feeling the pull along your left side.
- Repeat with the right arm, then the left.
- Now stand with your feet about 18 inches apart, toes still pointing toward the front. Continue with the arm stretch in this position, right, left, right, left, to the count of 4.
- Bring your feet together in their original side-by-side position and do 4 alternating stretches, then stand with your feet apart for 4 stretches.
- Repeat this combination until you have done 4 sets of stretches with your feet together and 4 sets with your feet apart.

Body Roll

Here's another warm-up stretch that can begin to stretch the muscles of the neck, back, and backs of the legs. (Don't do this exercise, or any exercise that causes a rush of blood to the head, if you are in the throes of a migraine or feel a migraine coming on.)

- Stand up straight with your feet about 18 inches apart. Roll the head forward attempting to touch the chin to the chest.
- Round the upper back and continue to roll forward, letting the arms hang toward the floor.
- Bend your knees as much as you need to feel comfortable as you continue to bend forward until you can touch the floor. (Palms flat on the floor is best, if you can safely and gently manage it. But don't go farther than you safely can.) Hold for a count of 4.

- Slowly roll upward, one vertebra at a time, until you once again stand straight. Keep your head down, chin toward the chest, until your body is completely erect. Then slowly raise it.
- Repeat: Slowly roll down to 4 counts, hold for 4 counts, then slowly rise for 4 counts. Do this exercise at least 6 times.

Upper Back Release

You may not realize how much tension you're carrying in your upper back until you do this exercise and feel the relief! It's also good for pulling back rounded shoulders. (Don't do this exercise, or any exercise that causes a rush of blood to the head, if you are in the throes of a migraine or feel a migraine coming on.)

- Stand straight, feet about 18 inches apart, facing straight ahead. Clasp your hands behind your back and straighten your arms. (You'll feel your shoulder blades being pinned together.)
- Bend forward at the waist, keeping your hands clasped and arms straight. Bend your knees and bring your head toward the floor as far as you can.
- Maintaining this position, pull your clasped hands and straight arms toward your head as much as possible. Hold to a count of 4.
- Slowly raise your body to a standing position, relaxing your arms back down toward your buttocks. (Keep hands clasped throughout.)
- Repeat this exercise 4 times.

BODY ALIGNMENT

Exercise can do a great deal to relieve the muscle tension that contributes to migraines. But standing and sitting correctly are also important parts of the equation. Poor posture can exert undue pressure on your neck, shoulder, and back muscles and nerves, leading to headaches. Too many people round their shoulders, hunch their upper backs, and jut their heads and necks forward, irritating muscles and nerves. Our modern lifestyle doesn't help. Sitting at a computer all day, holding the phone between your shoulder and cheek, or even pressing your cell phone to your ear can increase muscle tension and throw your neck and spine out of alignment.

Because of this, it seems worthwhile to go over the principles of good posture, beginning at the top of the body. Well, almost. I like to start with the shoulders rather than the head, because most people carry their heads in the wrong position. If we start with an improperly positioned head, and go from there, then where are we? But the shoulders can show us just where the head should sit.

In Good Standing

With that in mind, raise your shoulders and roll them back to the point where your chest juts out and your "wing bones" (scapulae) are pulled toward the center of your back. Then relax until you no longer feel your chest jutting out unnaturally but your shoulders aren't rounding and your chest is open, not collapsed. This is the correct position for your shoulders—neither yanked back nor rounded forward.

Now lift your head and pull your chin in toward your neck slightly. If an imaginary midline was drawn from the middle of the side of your neck to the top of your shoulders, your ears should sit directly above it. Your eyes should focus straight ahead at about horizon level, or slightly lower.

Once you've mastered this position of the head, neck, and shoulders, the rest should be easy. The main thing to remember is that most of us tend to sway our backs—that is, to release the buttocks toward the back and the stomach toward the front. This is very stressful to the muscles of the lower back and throws the entire body out of alignment. Contract both the stomach muscles and the buttocks. Then "roll the buttocks under"— that's the opposite of releasing them toward the back. Think of making the curve in your lower back less exaggerated. You'll find it easier to do this if you bend your knees just slightly. Locked knees encourage a swayed back and a protruding stomach.

To complete the ideal of a good standing posture, your knees should point straight forward and your feet should point forward also, angled just slightly outward, or away from each other. (The opposite is "pigeon-toed.") Don't angle feet too far outward, though. Think of the hands of a clock: If your heels were positioned at 6, the left foot would point toward 11 and the right one toward 1. Keep your weight mostly on the balls of your feet, with less on the outside edges and heels. (Don't roll your weight toward the inner edge of your foot toward your arch. This will also throw off your alignment.)

Sitting Pretty

When you're sitting, the correct position of your upper body is essentially the same as when standing. Keep in mind that we all spend a great deal of time with our heads angled forward looking downward—a stressful position for the neck. We look down to read, to write, to cook, to take care of our children, to shop, to garden, and to do housework. Whenever possible, try to accomplish your aims by looking straight ahead, as if looking at the horizon or slightly below it. Position your computer screen so that it's at eye level. Hold up your book or newspaper, use document holders when typing, and position frequently used items on eye-level shelves. Naturally, there are still plenty of things that can't be raised to horizon level for the convenience of your neck. But you can develop an awareness of how often you look down, then take frequent breaks from such activity. Get up from your desk, stretch, walk around, and change activities often. For many people, just rearranging their workstations can make a big difference in the amount of neck and shoulder stress they endure daily.

PUTTING IT ALL TOGETHER

Your physical strategies for migraine prevention should include the following:

- Maintain good posture when standing or sitting.
- Take frequent stretching breaks from your desk or computer to avoid the accumulation of muscle tension.
- Get at least thirty minutes of moderately intensive exercise per day.
- Do back and neck stretches daily.
- Don't exercise while in the throes of a headache.

And remember: Check with your physician before beginning, intensifying, or changing your exercise or activity regimen. It's best to be safe.

Chapter 10

——◀◯▶——

If Medicine Is Necessary

Migraines have been with us for so long that we really can't say when they first began plaguing mankind. Naturally, a good many treatments have been devised throughout the ages, including stuffing a little piece of an herb into a slit cut into the skin of the forehead. Holding a burning-hot piece of metal to the painful part of the head was also tried. This "medicine" probably wouldn't reverse the brain changes that caused the migraine, but it would certainly distract one from the original pain!

Despite the inventiveness of early healers, it wasn't until the middle of the twentieth century that the first specific—and safe—migraine treatment was devised. During the 1940s, a drug called *ergotamine tartrate,* or *ergot,* was introduced. Up until then, migraineurs had been forced to rely on "general" medicines such as painkillers. But this new drug, the first treatment specially targeted to migraines, helped quite a few people by working through the serotonin system to restore blood vessels in the head to their normal size. Unfortunately, it wasn't a very selective drug; that is, it affected various serotonin receptors, not just the ones responsible for migraines. As a result, it touched off some very unpleasant side effects, including nausea and vomiting. In addition, ergot wasn't very ambitious. It relieved the pain, but left other migraine symptoms alone. To make matters worse, some patients became dependent on the drug: They *had* to keep taking it.

Ergot was joined in the 1950s by *dihydroergotamine mesylate,* or DHE. A cousin of the earlier drug, DHE also triggered some unpleasant side effects, including nausea in up to half of its users. And like ergot, DHE did not help with the nonpain symptoms of migraine.

And so migraineurs only had limited choices. There were two migraine-specific drugs that helped with pain but not with other migraine symptoms, and caused side effects. Sufferers could also choose from a variety of painkillers and other medicines that helped some people, to some degree. In short, we doctors could help many patients a little bit, and a few patients quite a bit. But we didn't have that "magic pill" in our pharmacopoeia, the medicine that could quickly knock out migraine pain in most people, relieve the other symptoms as well, and not produce unpalatable side effects. And as for preventing future migraines, well, that appeared to be a pipe dream.

A new era in the drug treatment of migraines began in the early 1990s, when *Imitrex* (known by the generic name of *sumatriptan succinate*) joined the antimigraine arsenal. A more discriminating drug, it selectively targets certain receptor sites in the body. It's like the "smart bombs" that home in on specific targets, rather than exploding on anything they happen to contact. With this and other new drugs, we doctors finally had a reasonable array of medicines to offer our patients. At last, we could help stop migraines in progress, manage some of the symptoms associated with migraines, and possibly ward off new attacks.

Why is this important? Why are we even talking about drugs, when this book is dedicated to introducing my all-natural triple therapy? There are three reasons. First, the triple therapy works best for those who have low levels of magnesium and/or riboflavin. There are many other migraineurs who have good levels of these nutrients, and/or may not respond well to feverfew. Thus they may not be helped by the triple therapy. Second, even when you're on the triple therapy, you may still be hit by migraines. Most of my patients report "far fewer migraines," "a real big drop in attacks," and "hardly any more." That's a tremendous achievement, but it's not perfect—some migraines still manage to sneak through. Finally, it may take a little while for the triple therapy to become fully effective, so you may need some medicines in the meantime.

Trade and Generic Names

Drug names give most people problems because each drug has so many of them.

First there's the *chemical name,* the barely pronounceable word that describes the drug's chemical formulation. For example, 3-{2-(dimethylamino)ethyl}-N-methyl-indole-5-methanesulfonamide is the chemical name for Imitrex.

Then there's the *generic name,* the medicine's official name that tells you something about the drug. For example, just by looking at the generic name naratriptan you can tell the drug is a member of the triptan family of drugs. You can easily identify generic names because they're not capitalized, are not followed by the little ® that indicates that it's a registered and protected name, and are usually uninspiring.

Finally, there's the *trade name*. This is the registered name given to a drug by its manufacturer. Inderal, Imitrex, and Excedrin are all trade names. Trade names are capitalized and are often followed by the ® that indicates the name is registered. Plus, they're usually easier to pronounce than the generic names. More and more, in fact, trade names are designed with marketing in mind, so they're flashy-sounding or they tell you what they do. For example, the name Procardia tells you that the drug does something positive ("pro") for the heart ("cardia"), and the name Glucotrol makes it clear that this drug controls ("cotrol") blood sugar or glucose ("glu") and helps diabetics.

If you don't mind stretching the explanation a little bit, think of how the three types of names would be applied to a common household item. "Plasticized-humanoidrepresentation" would be the item's chemical name, "doll" the generic name, and the trade name would be "Barbie."

We'll give both trade and generic names in the discussion of drugs that follows. Generic names will be in parentheses.

MEDICINE FOR MIGRAINES

There are many drugs in our antimigraine arsenal, ranging from those that attack the pain to those that handle the side effects, from those designed specifically for migraines to those that were developed for other diseases but turned out to be helpful for migraineurs. The numerous types of drugs fall into two larger categories: *abortive* drugs to stop migraines in progress, and *prophylactic* drugs to prevent future ones from striking.

Abortive Drugs

- *Corticosteroids.* Prednisone and other corticosteroids work by dampening the body's inflammation response. They're generally used for very long-lasting migraines that don't respond to other treatments. Side effects include insomnia, anxiety, and agitation. Depending on the drug, the corticosteroids may be given orally or via injection. These drugs have a large number of serious side effects if used for long periods of time.
- *Ergot derivatives.* Cafergot, Migranal, Ercaf, and other drugs in this family are derived from a plant fungus. They are felt to help with migraines by constricting the blood vessels in the brain (and, unfortunately, elsewhere). Their potential side effects include nausea, vomiting, and muscle cramps. Depending on the drug, they can be taken orally, sublingually, via injection, or as a suppository.
- *Opioids or narcotics.* Percocet (oxycodone with acetaminophen), Vicodin (hydrocodone with acetaminophen), Demerol (meperidine), and other power painkillers are used for more serious migraines that don't respond to first-line medical therapy. Side effects include dizziness, sedation,

vomiting, irritability, and perspiration. There's also the very real danger of dependency and addiction.

- *NSAIDs.* These are the nonsteroidal anti-inflammatory drugs prescribed for arthritis and many other painful ailments. Advil (ibuprofen), Motrin (ibuprofen), Naprosyn (naproxen), Relafen (nabumetone) and other NSAIDs, plus over-the-counter versions of plain old aspirin, have long been used for migraines. Potential side effects of these over-the-counter and prescription drugs include urinary tract infections, diarrhea, nausea, and stomach bleeding.

- *Triptans.* A relatively new treatment for migraines, the triptans work by encouraging the action of the neurotransmitter serotonin. Depending on the drug, they can be taken orally, via nasal spray and/or via an injection. Potential side effects of the triptans include feeling warm, muscle weakness, shortness of breath, chest pain, and anxiety. If you have heart disease, or risk factors for heart disease, taking triptans can be dangerous because they can cause coronary arteries that are already narrowed to constrict even more, possibly triggering a heart attack. Amerge, Imitrex, Maxalt, and Zomig are members of this family of medicines.

- *Combination drugs.* These include Fiorinal (butalbital, caffeine, and aspirin), Fioricet and Esgic (butalbital, caffeine, and acetaminophen), and Midrin (isometheptene, dichloralphenazone, and acetaminophen). Potential side effects include somnolence, worsening of headaches with frequent use, and, with the exception of Midrin, dependency and addiction.

Prophylactic Drugs

- *Antidepressants.* Elavil (amitriptyline), Pamelor (nortriptyline), and similar drugs are intended to treat depression, but they can also help with migraines. These medicines possess painkilling properties and relieve most types of chronic pain, probably through the serotonin system. Potential side effects include dry mouth, constipation, somnolence, anxiety, irregular heartbeat, elevated blood pressure, and weight gain.

- *Antiseizure medications.* Odd as it sounds, Depakote (divalproex sodium), as well as other medicines designed to prevent seizures, have been used to prevent migraines. The reasoning is that excessive excitation of certain nerve cells leads to a seizure, while excitation of cells in a different area triggers a migraine. These drugs suppress excessive excitation of all brain cells. Potential side effects include weight gain, loss of hair, bruising, nausea, and potential damage to the liver or pancreas. Neurontin (gabapentin) and Topamax (topiramate) are other anticonvulsants being used for the treatment of pain and migraine headaches, with fewer side effects.

- *Beta-blockers.* Inderal (propranolol), Lopressor (metoprolol), Blocadren (timolol), and other members of this family of drugs are perhaps best known to the general public as medicines for certain heart problems and elevated blood pressure. The beta-blockers help to relax blood vessels, and interfere with the catecholamine hormones that attempt to make the vessels squeeze down again. Potential side effects include dizziness, slow heartbeat, depression, and fatigue. They cannot be used in patients with a history of asthma. Also known as beta-adrenergic blocking agents and beta-blocking agents, these drugs are commonly prescribed for migraines.

- *Calcium channel blockers.* Like the beta-blockers, these were designed to treat elevated blood pressure and heart problems. These drugs work by interfering with calcium, which constricts blood vessels. Unfortunately, Calan (verapamil) and other calcium channel blockers are not very effective and have side effects such as constipation, congestive heart failure, fluid retention, shortness of breath, blurred vision, flushing, and impotence.

- *MAO inhibitors.* Nardil (phenelzine) and other members of this family of drugs are primarily intended to treat depression. They're also used for migraines, especially severe attacks, and for chronic daily headaches. Unfortunately, the MAO inhibitors can cause a lot of unwanted side effects, including weight gain, dry mouth, insomnia, and constipation, while an overdose may lead to tremor, manic behavior, and other problems. Since these drugs can interact with a large number of foods and drugs, patients should be given a detailed list of instructions for safe usage.

- *Botox* (Botulinum toxin type A) was originally developed for the treatment of involuntary forceful blinking. Then it was noticed that wrinkles around the eyes of people treated with Botox flattened out, and Botox became widely used for wrinkles in the forehead and elsewhere. This in turn led to the observation that migraines improved in many migraineurs getting the toxin. Like many of the other prophylactic drugs mentioned in this chapter, Botox is not approved for migraines, but I find it effective for up to 70 percent of patients with migraine headaches. The benefits of one treatment can last for three months.

A FEW BASIC RULES FOR PRESCRIBING

There's a basic rule I like to adhere to: Whenever possible, use the least potent medicine, and use as little as possible to accomplish the task. I'm not knocking drugs; they're often very helpful, and sometimes absolutely necessary. But as a medical doctor who has been observing the effects of drugs for two decades now, I can tell you that they all have side effects—sometimes serious ones. One day we'll undoubtedly have perfect drugs that erase pain without affecting anything else in the body. Until then, it's best to use these substances as sparingly as possible—enough to get the job done, but never more than needed, and never more powerful drugs than needed.

Just as we physicians try to limit the drugs prescribed, it's best if you use what you're given and nothing more. Only use drugs that have been prescribed for you by your physician, and only in the indicated amounts. Never use someone else's medicine, even if they have the same ailment you do. The fact that you and your friend both have migraines, for example, doesn't mean you should use the same dosage of the same drug. What may work very well for her may be useless for you—or worse, harmful.

It doesn't matter if you and your friends are the same height, weight, body type, age, and so on: You can still have different body chemistries and very different medicinal needs. It doesn't even matter if we're talking about your sister, with whom you share a lot of genes. Body chemistry is very individual, which means that the selection of the right drug for you is also a very individual matter.

For pregnant and nursing women, caution is always the rule. Anything you take might affect your baby, so it's very important that you and your physician weigh all the alternatives very carefully and try to avoid drugs as much as possible. Even nonprescription items you pick up in the drugstore or supermarket should be used as sparingly as possible, and only after you've talked with your physician about them.

Be sure to give your doctor a complete list of all the drugs you take—even over-the-counter items you bought in the drugstore or supermarket. There are a great many drug-to-drug interactions that can change the way a medicine works in your body, so be sure to tell your physician about *all* the medicines you're taking. Let him or her know about any supplements you take as well.

A note about children: Many of the drugs used by adults have not been tested on children. Even though some of these should theoretically be safe and helpful for children, it's best to exercise the utmost caution when prescribing for youngsters. If your child has migraines, be sure to work with a physician experienced in treating children who is attuned to their special needs.

The same holds true for seniors. We really don't know if many of the migraine medicines are suited for people over the age of sixty-five. Theoretically, there's no reason why a pill should be helpful up until your sixty-fifth birthday, then become useless. But remember that seniors often have multiple health problems, multiple health risks, and are taking multiple drugs. They may be more susceptible to drug side effects just because their bodies are not functioning quite as well as they were in years past. Until a drug is proven safe for senior citizens, we should approach it with caution.

When trying prophylactic drugs, it is important to start with a low dose, then escalate the dose to the level where it either provides relief or causes side effects. A common mistake is for a patient (and sometimes a doctor) to try a small dose of a particular drug (such as 10 mg of Elavil or 60 mg of Inderal) and, if it is ineffective at that dosage, to move on to another drug before giving the first drug a full trial.

Now let's take a look at some of the migraine medicines. For the sake of convenience, I've divided them into several categories: medicines for attacks in progress, medicines to prevent future attacks, and medicines for the other symptoms of migraines.

Alerted, Not Frightened Away

As you read through the descriptions of the drugs that follow, you'll notice I list some of the potential side effects, mention some of the people who should *not* take the drugs, and point to a few of the possible drug-to-drug interactions you may encounter.

I'm not trying to scare you away from drugs; I'm not suggesting that you should never take them. Rather, I want you to be aware of the possible problems you may encounter when taking these—or any other—medications. I want to alert you to potential danger so you'll have a thorough discussion with your physician about the pros and cons of each drug as the two of you decide what's best for you.

Don't let your doctor get away with simply handing you a prescription. Make sure he or she reviews your needs, medical history, and personal history thoroughly, and carefully explains how to use the medicine.

SOME MEDICINES FOR
ATTACKS IN PROGRESS

These drugs, known as abortives, are designed to relieve headaches in progress. They do not prevent future headaches or make them less severe.

Medicines to stop migraines in progress range from over-the-counter capsules to those powerful drugs that must be injected in a doctor's office. If you have relatively mild migraines, Advil Migraine (identical to Advil Liqui-Gels, and both faster in action than plain Advil), Excedrin Migraine (identical to Excedrin), Aleve (naproxen sodium), ibuprofen, or another non-prescription medicine may be all you need. Although over-the-counter drugs are generally milder than their prescription cousins, they can be dangerous: Gastrointestinal distress is a common side effect. If you use these or similar medicines for your migraines, be sure to review your dosage with your physician. And be sure to tell your doctor if you're using over-the-counter medications *in addition* to prescription medicines.

Below you'll find a brief overview of the major prescription abortives. These are not all of the drugs that may be used, and the description of each is not meant to be complete. Rather, this section is designed to give you an idea of how each medicine is used and some of the things you should consider before taking it. I urge you to discuss each drug thoroughly with your physician before taking it. Be sure to review the side effects and reasons why you should or should not use it with your doctor, and make sure you understand the dosage instructions.

And remember, these drugs are meant to help with a migraine in progress, not prevent future ones.

This discussion of abortive drugs is geared for adults under the age of sixty-five. Children and seniors over the age of sixty-five have special needs.

Amerge (naratriptan)

Amerge, available in the U.S. since 1998, is the longest-acting of the triptans. It's also a relatively slow-acting medicine.

Which types of migraines is it for? With or without aura. It may be helpful in menstrual migraines.

When is it taken? When you first notice the symptoms of a migraine.

How much is in a usual dose? 1.0–2.5 mg.

What's the maximum I should take? 5 mg per day is considered the maximum that should be taken.

What happens if I take too much? You'll suffer from the side effects, but in a more pronounced way.

What side effects should I watch for? Potential side effects include nausea, dizziness, drowsiness, pins-and-needles sensations, throat tightness, and fatigue.

Who should not *take this drug, or be very cautious about doing so?* This drug should not be used by anyone with angina, a previous heart attack, other heart or circulatory problems, high blood pressure, or liver or kidney disease. Pregnant and nursing women should approach this medicine with extreme caution.

Are there other drugs that should not be taken while using Amerge? This drug should not be used if you are taking ergot-type medications, or if you've taken another triptan (Imitrex, Maxaltz, or Zomig) the same day you intend to take Amerge. Be sure to let your doctor know about all the medications you're taking.

Cafergot

Cafergot contains ergotamine tartrate and caffeine. That's easy to remember if you look at the drug's name: think of "caf" as representing caffeine, with "ergot" standing for ergotamine. Cafergot is available as a tablet and a suppository. Both the ergotamine and the caffeine help constrict the blood vessels in the brain.

Which types of migraines is it for? With or without aura.

When is it taken? When you first notice the symptoms of a migraine.

How much is in a usual dose? One tablet is the standard dose for tablets. For suppositories, half or even a quarter of a suppository can provide relief without side effects, while a whole suppository may worsen nausea.

What's the maximum I should take? 3 tablets or suppositories in 24 hours.

What happens if I take too much? Using too much Cafergot, or any other ergotamine-containing medicine, may cause headaches, convulsions, elevated or weakened blood pressure, vomiting, muscle pain, and numbness. You may feel cold, and your fingers and toes may become pale. Untreated, ergot poisoning can lead to gangrene and amputation. It's also possible to become psychologically dependent on the medicine, especially if you've been taking it for a long time.

What side effects should I watch for? Potential side effects include elevated blood pressure, numbness, nausea, vomiting, a rapid or slow heartbeat, and weakness. And because the drug causes blood vessels to constrict ("squeeze down"), it may interfere with the flow of blood. This can cause chest pain, and the skin may turn bluish. You may also feel cold and your muscles may hurt.

Who should not *take this drug, or be very cautious about doing so?* Anyone who has suffered an allergic reaction to drugs containing ergotamine, or to caffeine, should not use Cafergot. Those with high blood pressure, heart disease, problems with circulation, infections, or liver or kidney disease should also avoid its use. Pregnant and nursing women should not take this medicine.

Are there other drugs that should not be taken while using Cafergot? Taking it with Sudafed or other drugs that cause blood vessels to constrict may be dangerous. Other drugs, including Nicoderm and other nicotine drugs, beta-blockers such as Inderal, and antibiotics may interfere with the way Cafergot works in the body. Be sure to let your doctor know about all the medications you're taking.

Demerol (meperidine hydrochloride)

This is a very popular opioid or narcotic analgesic.

Which types of migraines is it for? Severe attacks that do not respond to other migraine drugs, when other drugs are contraindicated or are not tolerated.

When is it taken? When you first notice the symptoms of a migraine.

How much is in a usual dose? 25–100 mg in an injection, or 100–400 mg in tablet form.

What's the maximum I should take? 300 mg in injection and 1200 mg in oral form, but if these amounts are taken for several days in a row an epileptic seizure may occur.

What happens if I take too much? Symptoms of an overdose include cold and clammy skin, muscle weakness, difficulty breathing, and coma. Use with caution, for it is possible to become mentally and physically dependent on this drug.

What side effects should I watch for? Potential side effects include nausea, sweating, vomiting, and sleepiness.

Who should not *take this drug, or be very cautious about doing so?* There's a long list of people who should avoid or be very careful with this drug, including those with liver disease, kidney disease, an underactive thyroid, Addison's disease, an enlarged prostate and irregular heartbeat. Pregnant and nursing women should approach this medicine with extreme caution.

Are there other drugs that should not be taken while using Demerol? MAO inhibitors should not be taken while you're on this drug. Demerol can interfere with the action of many drugs in your body, including antihistamines, tranquilizers, and antidepressants. Be sure to let your doctor know about all the medications you're taking.

DHE-45

This is the abbreviation for dihydroergotamine, which is usually given in an intravenous or intramuscular injection. DHE-45 has been given to many patients who stagger into their doctor's offices or emergency rooms in the throes of a migraine. It can be effective when a prolonged migraine, or so-called migraine status, occurs. DHE-45 can be given in a 1 mg dose every 8 hours intravenously for several days to break a prolonged attack. For more on DHE-45, skip down a few items to Migranal, a form of DHE-45 that comes as a nasal spray.

Ergomar (ergotamine tartrate) sublingual tablet

This drug belongs to the ergot family.

Which types of migraines is it for? With and without aura.

When is it taken? When you first notice the symptoms of a migraine.

How much is in a usual dose? One 2 mg tablet taken under the tongue.

What's the maximum I should take? 4 tablets a day.

What happens if I take too much? You risk the same problems as you do if you take too much Cafergot.

What side effects should I watch for? Potential side effects are the same as you can expect to see with Cafergot.

Who should not *take this drug, or be very cautious about doing so?* Pregnant and nursing women cannot take it—can cause miscarriage in pregnant women.

Are there other drugs that should not be taken while using Ergomar? Triptans should not be taken. Be sure to let your doctor know about all the medications you're taking.

Fioricet

This is one of the "3 fees": Fioricet, Fiorinal, and Fiorinal with Codeine. These are a group of related drugs containing caffeine, a sedative barbiturate called butalbital, plus an NSAID. And of course, Fiorinal with Codeine also contains a narcotic.

Fioricet, the first of the "3 fees" we'll look at, consists of caffeine, butalbital, and acetaminophen. It's also found under the brand names of Anolor 300, Esgic, and Esgic-Plus. The difference between this drug and Fiorinal is that instead of aspirin this drug contains acetaminophen, which is *not* a form of aspirin.

Which types of migraines is it for? It is approved for tension headaches, but is used for migraines with and without aura.

When is it taken? When you first notice the symptoms of a migraine.

How much is a usual dose? 1 tablet, which contains a standard mixture of 50 mg butalbital, 40 mg caffeine, and 325 mg acetaminophen.

What's the maximum I should take? 4 tablets a day.

What happens if I take too much? An overdose can produce a variety of symptoms, including confusion, drowsiness, excess perspiration, nausea, shock, and coma. Because this drug contains a barbiturate, taking too much can lead to physical and mental dependence. Taking it on a regular basis causes worsening of headaches—what's known as the rebound effect.

What side effects should I watch for? Potential side effects include pain in the abdomen, drowsiness, feeling intoxicated, nausea, shortness of breath, and vomiting.

Who should not *take this drug, or be very cautious about doing so?* Those who have had reactions to caffeine, acetaminophen, or barbiturates should avoid this drug, as should anyone who has the metabolic disorder known as porphyria, liver disease, kidney disease, or abdominal distress. Those who have trouble with drug abuse, or who are or have been severely depressed, should let their doctors know before taking this medicine. Pregnant and nursing women should approach this medicine with extreme caution.

Are there other drugs that should not be taken while using Fioricet? This drug can interfere with the action of several drugs in your body, including antihistamines, antidepressants, muscle relaxants, narcotics, and tranquilizers. Be sure to let your doctor know about all the medications you're taking.

Fiorinal

The second of the "3 fees," Fiorinal is just like Fioricet, but instead of acetaminophen it has aspirin to go with the caffeine and butalbital. It's also found under the trade name of Isollyl.

Which types of migraines is it for? It is approved for tension headaches, but is used for migraines with and without aura.

When is it taken? When you first notice the symptoms of a migraine.

How much is in a usual dose? 1 tablet.

What's the maximum I should take? 4 tablets a day.

What happens if I take too much? An overdose can lead to delirium, fever, insomnia, irregular heartbeat, seizures, vomiting, and other problems. Because this drug contains a barbiturate, taking too much can lead to physical and mental dependence.

What side effects should I watch for? Potential side effects are dizziness, drowsiness, nausea, vomiting, and gas.

Who should not *take this drug, or be very cautious about doing so?* Those who have had reactions to caffeine, aspirin, or barbiturates should avoid this drug, as should anyone who has the metabolic disorder known as porphyria. Fiorinal contains aspirin, so it should not be given to children and teenagers with the flu or chicken pox (it may lead to Reye's syndrome). The aspirin also makes this drug potentially dangerous for anyone with problems with blood-clotting or bleeding problems, or ulcers. Anyone with liver disease, kidney disease, intestinal ailments, an enlarged prostate, a head injury, thyroid problems, or urinary disorders should be cautious. Those who have trouble with drug abuse, or who are or have been severely depressed should let their doctors know before taking this medicine. Pregnant and nursing women should approach this medicine with extreme caution.

Are there other drugs that should not be taken while using Fiorinal? This drug can interfere with the actions of a variety of other drugs in the body, including beta-blockers, MAO inhibitors, the arthritis drug Rheumatrex, narcotic pain relievers, oral contraceptives, and tranquilizers. Be sure to let your doctor know about all the medications you're taking.

Fiorinal with Codeine

Fiorinal with Codeine has the same caffeine, butalbital, and aspirin found in Fiorinal, plus codeine phosphate. It's considered a strong narcotic painkiller.

Which types of migraines is it for? It is approved for tension headaches, but is used for migraines with and without aura.

When is it taken? When you first notice the symptoms of a migraine.

How much is in a usual dose? 1 tablet.

What's the maximum I should take? 4 tablets a day.

What happens if I take too much? Signs of an overdose include confusion, low blood pressure, difficulty breathing, shock, and coma. Because this drug contains a barbiturate, taking too much can lead to physical and mental dependence.

What side effects should I watch for? Potential side effects include drowsiness, dizziness, elevated blood sugar, irritability, and abdominal pain.

Who should not *take this drug, or be very cautious about doing so?* Those who have had reactions to caffeine, aspirin, or barbiturates should avoid this drug, as should anyone who has the metabolic disorder known as porphyria. Fiorinal contains aspirin, so it should not be given to children and teenagers with the flu or chicken pox (it may lead to Reye's syndrome). The aspirin also makes this drug potentially dangerous for anyone with blood-clotting problems or bleeding problems, a vitamin K deficiency, nasal polyps, fluid retention, or ulcers. Anyone with liver disease, kidney disease, intestinal ailments, an enlarged prostate, a head injury, thyroid problems, or urinary disorders should be cautious. Those who have trouble with drug abuse, or who are or have been severely depressed should let their doctors know before taking this medicine. Pregnant and nursing women should approach this medicine with extreme caution.

Are there other drugs that should not be taken while using Fiorinal with Codeine? This drug can interfere with the action of many other medicines in the body, including antidepressants, antigout drugs, antihistamines, beta-blockers, blood thinners, insulin, NSAIDs, oral contraceptives, and tranquilizers. Be sure to let your doctor know about all the medications you're taking.

Imitrex (sumatriptan succinate)

This popular migraine medicine can be taken as an injection, a tablet, or a nasal spray. It's considered the "gold standard" for stopping migraines that hit hard and fast. It's also used for cluster headaches.

Which types of migraines is it for? An acute migraine, with or without aura. It is *not* used for basilar and hemiplegic migraines.

When is it taken? When you first notice the symptoms of a migraine.

How much is in a usual dose? If you're taking it in tablet form, 50 mg is a standard dose; 100 mg is considered the most you should take at any one time. Your doctor *may* instruct you to take a second dose if the first does not work. Your doctor may also give you permission to take a second dose a couple of hours later if the headache returns. As a nasal spray, Imitrex comes in 5 mg and 20 mg doses. As an injection, it comes in a 6 mg dose that can be self-injected with a penlike device.

What's the maximum I should take? 200 mg in tablet form is considered the maximum dose per day. Two doses of the nasal spray (40 mg) or two injections (12 mg) are the maximum per day.

What happens if I take too much? Some signs of overdose are poor coordination, a feeling of sluggishness, tremor, the skin developing a bluish tinge, and convulsions.

What side effects should I watch for? Potential side effects include dizziness, feelings of heaviness or tightness, muscle weakness, pain and stiffness in the neck, a sore throat, and a feeling of being warm. Some less common side effects are a severe allergic reaction to the drug, anxiety and agitation, difficulty urinating, headaches, itching, muscle pain, a feeling of pressure in the chest, shortness of breath, sweating, and the "blahs."

Who should not *take this drug, or be very cautious about doing so?* Those with angina, previous heart attacks, or certain other heart problems, as well as people with high blood pressure, liver disease, or peripheral vascular disease. Pregnant and nursing women should approach this medicine with extreme caution.

Are there other drugs that should not be taken while using Imitrex? Any drugs with ergotamine should not be taken while you're using Imitrex. You should also avoid Sansert and certain other medications such as Nardil and other MAO inhibitors. Prozac, Zoloft, and other SSRIs (selective serotonin re-uptake inhibitors) can, in rare instances, interact with Imitrex and other triptans to cause very unpleasant and serious reactions. However, the vast majority of patients can take an SSRI like Zoloft together with Imitrex without any interaction. You should not use this drug if you've taken another triptan (Amerge, Maxalt, or Zomig) the same day. Be sure to let your doctor know about all the medications you're taking.

Maxalt (rizatriptan benzoate)

Another of the triptans, Maxalt "melts in the mouth," which means it can be taken without water. Actually, the drug comes in two forms, Maxalt and Maxalt-MLT. It's the latter that is broken down by saliva. Both work rapidly.

Which types of migraines is it for? With and without aura.

When is it taken? When you first notice the symptoms of a migraine.

How much is in a usual dose? 10 mg.

What's the maximum I should take? 30 mg a day.

What happens if I take too much? You'll suffer from the same types of problems you would if you took too much Imitrex.

What side effects should I watch for? Potential side effects include sleepiness, fatigue, dizziness, and pain or pressure in the throat or chest.

Who should not *take this drug, or be very cautious about doing so?* Anyone with heart disease or a history of heart disease, or elevated blood pressure. Pregnant and nursing women should approach this medicine with extreme caution.

Are there other drugs that should not be taken while using Maxalt? You should not use this drug if you've taken an MAO inhibitor within the past two weeks, or another triptan (Amerge, Imitrex, or Zomig) or an ergotamine-type drug within the past 24 hours.

Be sure to let your doctor know about all the medications you're taking.

Midrin

Midrin contains isometheptene mucate, dichloralphenazone, and acetaminophen.

Which types of headaches is it for? Migraines, tension and other types of headaches.

When is it taken? When you first notice the symptoms of a migraine.

How much is in a usual dose? 2 capsules followed by 1 every hour as needed.

What's the maximum I should take? 5 capsules a day.

What happens if I take too much? You'll feel drowsy and dizzy.

What side effects should I watch for? Potential side effects include dizziness and rash.

Who should not take this drug, or be very cautious about doing so? Anyone with glaucoma, heart problems, liver or kidney disease, elevated blood pressure, as well as those who have had a heart attack, stroke, or other problem involving the blood vessels. Pregnant and nursing women should approach this medicine with extreme caution.

Are there other drugs that should not be taken while using Midrin? You should avoid Midrin if you're taking Nardil or other MAO inhibitors. Other drugs—including Tylenol and others containing acetaminophen, antihistamines, and Valium or other central nervous system depressants—can change the way Midrin works in your body. Be sure to let your doctor know about all the medications you're taking.

Migranal (dihydroergotamine mesylate)

Migranal is an ergotamine-containing nasal spray that works by altering the amounts of serotonin in the brain.

Which types of migraines is it for? With or without aura. It's designed for people who need multiple doses of medicine for migraines that "come back." It's not meant for those with basilar or hemiplegic migraines.

When is it taken? When you first notice the symptoms of a migraine.

How much is in a usual dose? One packet of Migranal contains four doses of 0.5 mg each. Patients are typically instructed to spray one dose in each nostril, wait 15 minutes, then spray a second dose in each nostril. This comes to a total of 2 mg. Dosages for children and adults over the age of sixty-five have not been determined.

What's the maximum I should take? 4 mg per day is felt to be the maximum allowable dosage.

What happens if I take too much? Since Migranal contains a form of ergotamine, excessive intake can cause ergot poisoning symptoms such as headaches, convulsions, elevated or weakened blood pressure, vomiting, muscle pain, and numbness. You may feel cold, and your fingers and toes may become pale. Untreated, ergot poisoning can lead to gangrene and amputation.

What side effects should I watch for? Potential side effects include nausea, vomiting, dizziness, an altered sense of taste, and nasal distress. Elevated blood pressure, irregular heart rhythms, and heart attack are possible. Other potential side effects include swelling, itching, rash, cold and clammy skin, muscle weakness, confusion, increased sweating, and abdominal pain.

Who should not *take this drug, or be very cautious about doing so?* Migranal should not be used by anyone with infections, peripheral artery or heart disease, or liver or kidney disease. It is also contraindicated for those who have recently undergone vascular (blood vessel) surgery. Pregnant and nursing women should approach this medicine with extreme caution.

Are there other drugs that should not be taken while using Migranal? Vasoconstrictors such as Sansert (methysergide), triptans, and oral contraceptives may cause interactions or interfere with the way Migranal works in the body. Be sure to let your doctor know about all the medications you're taking.

Narcotics/Opioid Drug

Vicoprofen (hydrocodone with ibuprofen), Vicodin (hydrocodone with acetaminophen), Percocet (oxycodone with acetaminophen), Percodan (oxycodone with aspirin), and Stadol NS (butorphanol) are opioid (narcotic) analgesics that can relieve pain. Unfortunately, they often do *not* relieve other migraine symptoms. In fact, they can make nausea and other migraine symptoms worse. They also cause drowsiness: They may help relieve the pain, but you're not able to function. Other side effects of opioid drugs include constipation, confusion, and worsening of the headache. All the opioids carry risk of addiction as well as physical dependence if taken for prolonged periods of time.

I have a few patients who do not respond to or cannot tolerate other abortive medications and successfully treat their headaches with opioid drugs, but their number is very small. A very small number of people (about a dozen out of many thousands of my patients) can take a long-acting opioid drug, such as OxyContin (oxycodone, sustained release) or MS Contin (morphine, sustained release), for the prevention of headaches on a long-term basis.

Steroids

Prednisone (60 mg once, or for 2–3 days) is occasionally used to break an unusually severe attack. The injectable steroid Decadron (dexamethasone) can often stop an attack that does not respond to other treatments. (I first try a shot of magnesium, then a shot of Imitrex or D.H.E. 45, then Toradol, before moving on to steroids.)

Steroids are safe if taken once or twice a month, but long-term use is associated with many potential side effects, such as ulcers, hypertension, diabetes, osteoporosis, and bleeding.

Toradol (ketorolac)

Toradol is an NSAID used for moderately severe pain. It's not meant to be used for long periods of time.

Which types of migraines is it for? It's given to those who do not respond to oral medications.

When is it given? When other medications are ineffective.

How much is in a usual dose? You typically receive 30 to 60 mg of injectable Toradol. Tablets of this medication are available in 10 mg size, but in tablet form Toradol is not any stronger than ibuprofen or another NSAID—but it has more side effects.

What's the maximum I should take? If you do take tablets of Toradol, 40 mg is the maximum daily dose. This drug should not be used for more than 5 days total.

What happens if I take too much? You'll see the same problems as you would with other NSAIDs.

What side effects should I watch for? Potential side effects include dizziness, diarrhea, nausea, fluid retention, elevated blood pressure, itching, and sweating.

Who should not take this drug, or be very cautious about doing so? Anyone with peptic ulcer disease, kidney disease, liver disease, bleeding in the stomach or intestines, or other bleeding problems. Pregnant and nursing women should approach this medicine with extreme caution.

Are there other drugs that should not be taken while using Toradol? This drug should not be used if you're using aspirin, other NSAIDs, or probenecid. It can change the way many other drugs work in your body, including antidepressants, lithium, tranquilizers, Prozac, and other antidepressants. Be sure to let your doctor know about all the medications you're taking.

Zomig (zolmitriptan)

Zomig is a fast-acting triptan.

Which types of migraines is it for? With or without aura.

When is it taken? When you first notice the symptoms of a migraine.

How much is in a usual dose? For adults, 2.5 mg is the starting dose. That dose is adjusted to 5 mg as necessary. There is no widely accepted dose for children and adults over the age of sixty-five.

What's the maximum I should take? 10 mg per day. Your physician may give you the okay to take a second dose in the same day if your headache returns.

What happens if I take too much? You can expect to feel drowsy if you take too much. But don't let this relatively innocuous-sounding sign of overdose lull you into a false sense of security. Too much Zomig can cause other problems as well.

What side effects should I watch for? Potential side effects include pain, tightness or heaviness in the chest, pain or tightness in the jaw, neck, or throat, dizziness, feeling sleepy, dry mouth, weakness, and a sensation of being warm. Some of the less common side effects are muscle weakness or pain and difficulty swallowing. Zomig may also cause eye problems.

Who should not *take this drug, or be very cautious about doing so?* People with angina, past heart attacks, or other forms of heart disease; anyone with high blood pressure, or liver or kidney disease. Pregnant and nursing women should approach this medicine with extreme caution.

Are there other drugs that should not be taken while using Zomig? You should not use Zomig if you're on MAO inhibitors (such as Nardil or Parnate); if you've recently used Cafergot or other ergotamine-based migraine drugs; or if you're taking other triptans (Amerge, Imitrex, or Maxaltz). Other drugs, ranging from Tylenol to oral contraceptives, can interfere with the way Zomig works. Be sure to let your doctor know about all the medications you're taking.

SOME MEDICINES TO
PREVENT FUTURE ATTACKS

A fair number of drugs are used to prevent future attacks. They do help some people, but, unfortunately, they are a disappointment for many. Best estimates are that only half of the people taking preventive medications are helped to any significant degree.

Let's take a brief look at some of the more common drugs used to prevent migraines. These are not the only ones used, and the description of each is just a summary. The point is to give you an idea of how each medicine is used, as well as some of the things you should consider before taking it. I urge you to discuss each drug thoroughly with your physician before taking it. Be sure to review with your doctor the side effects and reasons why you should or should not use it, and make sure you understand the dosage instructions.

And remember, these drugs are meant to stop future migraines, not relieve ones that have already struck.

This discussion of preventive drugs is geared for adults under the age of sixty-five. Children and seniors over the age of sixty-five have special needs.

Calan (verapamil)

Verapamil is also available as Calan SR, Covera-HS, Isoptin, Isoptin SR, and Verelan.

What type of medicine is it? Verapamil is a calcium channel blocker used for heart and circulatory problems such as elevated blood pressure, irregular heartbeat, and angina.

How much is in a usual dose? 120 or 240 mg is a typical starting dose.

What's the maximum I should take? Some patients need up to 480 mg, and in rare cases higher doses.

What happens if I take too much? An overdose can cause blood pressure to fall dangerously low, and can trigger potentially fatal heart problems.

What side effects should I watch for? Potential side effects include heart failure, constipation, low blood pressure, cough, nausea, and rash.

Who should not *take this drug, or be very cautious about doing so?* Anyone with irregular heartbeat, low blood pressure, and certain other heart and circulatory problems; anyone who has had a bad reaction to this or other calcium channel blockers; those with liver or kidney disease; and people with a type of muscular dystrophy called Duchenne's. Pregnant and nursing women should approach this medicine with extreme caution.

Are there other drugs that should not be taken while using Calan? The drug can change the way other medicines act in your body, including ACE inhibitors, beta-blockers, alcohol, lithium, and Tagamet. Be sure to let your doctor know about all the medications you're taking.

Depakote (divalproex sodium)

This drug is available in a long-acting form called Depakote ER.

What type of medicine is it? Depakote is used to treat certain kinds of convulsions and seizures, plus the emotional fluctuations seen in manic-depressive disorder.

How much is in a usual dose? 250 mg per dose, two doses per day, is a common starting regimen or 500 mg once a day of the Depakote ER. The dosage may go as high as 2000 mg per day.

What's the maximum I should take? 2000 mg.

What happens if I take too much? An overdose can cause heart problems, make you feel very sleepy, and induce a coma. Be careful, for an overdose can be fatal.

What side effects should I watch for? Potential side effects include hair loss, weight gain, pain in the abdomen, difficulty breathing, constipation, diarrhea, dizziness, headache, insomnia, weakness, and tremor.

Who should not *take this drug, or be very cautious about doing so?* If you are allergic to the drug, or have liver problems, this drug is not for you. Depakote can make your blood "thinner" and less likely to clot, so it may be a problem for people who are already taking blood thinners or have clotting problems. It cannot be taken by pregnant women or women who are trying to conceive, for it can cause fetal malformations.

Are there other drugs that should not be taken while using Depakote? This medicine can interfere or enhance the action of several drugs, including aspirin, barbiturates, blood thinners, oral contraceptives, tranquilizers, and other seizure medicines. It can also make any alcohol you've consumed more potent. Be sure to let your doctor know about all the medications you're taking.

Elavil (amitriptyline hydrochloride)

What type of medicine is it? A tricyclic antidepressant used for depression, bulimia, and other problems.

How much is in a usual dose? They range from 10 mg to 100 mg, sometimes even higher. You and your physician may need to increase the dosage for several weeks before feeling any effect.

What's the maximum I should take? 100–200 mg.

What happens if I take too much? An overdose can cause dangerously low blood pressure, convulsions, confusion, hallucinations, problems with the heart, and coma.

What side effects should I watch for? Potential side effects include blurred vision, breast enlargement, confusion, constipation, increased perspiration, impotence, insomnia, hepatitis, and heart attack. Abruptly stopping the drug rather than tapering off can cause nausea, headaches, and other problems.

Who should not *take this drug, or be very cautious about doing so?* The elderly and those with heart trouble, glaucoma, or an enlarged prostate.

Are there other drugs that should not be taken while using Elavil? This drug should not be used if you're taking MAO inhibitors. Elavil can alter the way other drugs work in your body, including Sudafed, Prozac and other antidepressants, antihistamines, certain blood pressure medicines, and tranquilizers. Be sure to let your doctor know about all the medications you're taking.

Inderal (propranolol hydrochloride)

Inderal is also found as a long-acting Inderal LA.

What type of medicine is it? A beta-blocker commonly used for elevated blood pressure, angina, and certain other heart problems.

How much is in a usual dose? 80 mg per day. If 160–480 mg per day doesn't prevent migraines within a month or two, your doctor will wean you off this drug and switch you to a different medication.

What's the maximum I should take? 480 mg.

What happens if I take too much? An overdose may cause the heart to slow and become irregular, seizures, low blood pressure, and other serious problems.

What side effects should I watch for? Potential side effects include abdominal cramps, constipation, heart failure, depression, difficult breathing, low blood pressure, and slowing of the heartbeat.

Who should not *take this drug, or be very cautious about doing so?* People with poor circulation, slow or irregular heartbeat, asthma, heart failure, liver disease, kidney disease, or certain other problems should avoid Inderal. Pregnant and nursing women should approach this medicine with extreme caution.

Are there other drugs that should not be taken while using Inderal? This drug can alter the way many other drugs work in your body, including alcohol, insulin, calcium channel blockers, medicines for high blood pressure, NSAIDs, and oral diabetes drugs. Be sure to let your doctor know about all the medications you're taking.

Naprosyn (naproxen)

Naproxen is also available under the brand name EC-Naprosyn. Naprosyn, known generically as naproxen, is a close cousin to Anaprox, Aleve, and Naprelan, which are generically known as naproxen sodium.

What type of medicine is it? An NSAID used for arthritis, menstrual cramps, and other problems that produce mild to moderate pain.

How much is in a usual dose? 500 mg per day is a common starting dosage.

What's the maximum I should take? 1500 mg.

What happens if I take too much? An overdose can cause heartburn, nausea, vomiting, and drowsiness.

What side effects should I watch for? Potential side effects include peptic ulcers, gastrointestinal bleeding, difficulty breathing, abdominal pain, heartburn, nausea, and drowsiness.

Who should not *take this drug, or be very cautious about doing so?* Anyone who has had a reaction to this drug or related medicines such as Aleve, Anaprox, and EC-Naprosyn; those who have had bad reactions to aspirin or other NSAIDs; anyone with liver or kidney disease; and those taking blood thinners or who have blood-clotting problems.

Are there other drugs that should not be taken while using Naprosyn? Naprosyn can interfere with or alter the action of several drugs in your body, including aspirin, beta-blockers, blood thinners, methotrexate, oral diabetes drugs, and ACE inhibitors. Be sure to let your doctor know about all the medications you're taking.

Nardil (phenelzine sulfate)

This drug is not often used because of potential serious interactions with other medications and certain foods.

What type of medicine is it? An MAO (monoamine oxidase inhibitor) used for depression.

How much is in a usual dose? 15 mg, three times a day. If you and your doctor decide that you should stop taking Nardil, you'll be weaned off it rather than stopping it abruptly, for doing so can cause nightmares, convulsions, and other problems.

What's the maximum I should take? 90 mg.

What happens if I take too much? An overdose can cause numerous symptoms, including hallucinations, elevated blood pressure and body temperature, agitation, convulsions, and coma.

What side effects should I watch for? Potential side effects include dizziness, dry mouth, low blood pressure, sexual difficulties, and muscle spasms.

Who should not *take this drug, or be very cautious about doing so?* Anyone with heart failure, liver disease, an adrenal gland tumor known as pheochromocytoma, or diabetes. Pregnant and nursing women should approach this medicine with extreme caution.

Are there other drugs or other substances that should not be taken while using Nardil? A wide variety of drugs and other substances can interact with Nardil, including other MAO inhibitors, L-dopa, Prozac, and alcohol. Many foods can also interact with Nardil, including beer, certain cheeses, liver, wine, and yogurt. Be sure to let your doctor know about all the medications and supplements you're taking, and to review your diet with him or her.

Neurontin (gabapentin)

What type of medicine is it? An epilepsy drug designed to help with seizures.

How much is in a usual dose? Between 600 and 1800 mg per day.

What's the maximum I should take? 4800 mg.

What happens if I take too much? An overdose can cause slurred speech, double vision, drowsiness, and other problems.

What side effects should I watch for? Potential side effects include vision problems, fatigue, itchiness, poor muscular coordination, tremors, and nausea.

Who should not *take this drug, or be very cautious about doing so?* Anyone with liver or kidney diseases. Pregnant and nursing women should approach this medicine with extreme caution.

Are there other drugs that should not be taken while using Neurontin? This drug can interfere with the effects of antacids and other drugs in the body. Be sure to let your doctor know about all the medications you're taking.

Pamelor (nortriptyline hydrochloride)

This drug is very similar to amitriptyline, which is broken down in the body into nortriptyline, but has fewer side effects.

What type of medicine is it? A tricyclic antidepressant used for depression, and sometimes for chronic hives, bed-wetting, and other problems.

How much is in a usual dose? From 10 to 100 mg, sometimes higher. You and your physician may need to increase the dosage for several weeks before feeling any effect.

What's the maximum I should take? 100–200 mg.

What happens if I take too much? An overdose can cause problems with concentration, a very high fever, vomiting, a severe drop in blood pressure, shock, and stupor.

What side effects should I watch for? Potential side effects include blackening of the tongue, breast enlargement (even in men), dry mouth, fever, loss of appetite, nausea, heart problems, and ringing in the ears.

Who should not take this drug, or be very cautious about doing so? The elderly and those with heart trouble, glaucoma, or an enlarged prostate.

Are there other drugs that should not be taken while using Pamelor? This drug should not be used if you're taking MAO inhibitors, for the combination can be deadly. Pamelor can change the way certain drugs work in the body, including alcohol, drugs to open your airway, medicines for blood pressure and spasms, stimulants, and thyroid medications. Be sure to let your doctor know about all the medications you're taking.

Sansert (methysergide)

What type of medicine is it? It belongs to the ergot family.

How much is in a usual dose? 2 mg.

What's the maximum I should take? 12 mg.

What happens if I take too much? An overdose can cause the same kinds of problems you'd see with ergots such as Cafergot.

What side effects should I watch for? A rare but serious side effect after long-term use involves a thickening of tissue around the kidneys, heart, or lungs resulting in kidney, heart, or lung failure. This makes Sansert a drug of last resort.

Who should not *take this drug, or be very cautious about doing so?* Patients with circulatory problems. Pregnant and nursing women should not take this drug.

Are there other drugs that should not be taken while using Sansert? Be sure to let your doctor know about all the medications you're taking, so he or she can check for possible interactions.

Sinequan (doxepin hydrochloride)

What type of medicine is it? A tricyclic antidepressant used for depression, anxiety, and other problems.

How much is in a usual dose? 25 mg.

What's the maximum I should take? 100–200 mg.

What happens if I take too much? An overdose can cause a variety of symptoms, including confusion, agitation, dilated pupils, hallucinations, disturbances in body temperature, stupor, and coma.

What side effects should I watch for? Potential side effects include vision problems, confusion, constipation, diarrhea, hallucinations, and fever.

Who should not *take this drug, or be very cautious about doing so?* Anyone who has had a bad reaction to this or other antidepressants, plus anyone taking certain drugs that can combine dangerously with Sinequan in the body. Pregnant and nursing women should approach this medicine with extreme caution.

Are there other drugs that should not be taken while using Sinequan? Be sure to let your doctor know about all the medications you're taking, for mixing Sinequan with MAO inhibitors and certain other drugs can produce serious reactions, and may even be fatal. This drug can also change the way a host of other medicines work in the body, including antidepressants and tranquilizers.

SOME MEDICINES FOR THE OTHER SYMPTOMS OF MIGRAINES

Antinausea drugs (antiemetics) can sometimes relieve not just nausea, but some of the head pain as well. Triptans or another drug will relieve all kinds of symptoms in many patients, but many others are still left with nausea. And some people cannot take oral drugs because they throw up everything they attempt to swallow.

Taking an antiemetic in the form of a rectal suppository often stops the nausea and allows the patient to take an oral migraine drug. Phenergan (promethazine), Tigan (trimethobenzamide), Compazine (prochlorperazine), Reglan (metoclopramide), Thorazine (chlorpromazine), and Zofran (ondansetron) are some of the drugs we use for this purpose. The first three are available in a suppository form. The potential side effects include sedation, agitation, confusion and fatigue, and in some cases, involuntary movements of the body.

SOME QUESTIONS YOUR DOCTOR SHOULD ASK YOU BEFORE GIVING YOU ANY MEDICINE

All medicines, from aspirin to Zomig, have side effects. The medicine that works wonderfully for one person, without any noticeable side effects, may be worthless for you—or worse, deadly. That's why prescribing medications is a serious business, not to be taken lightly. Prescriptions should not be dashed off after just a few words with a patient. Instead, the person's needs, medical history, and family and personal history should be carefully reviewed. Your doctor should ask you these and many other questions before prescribing any medication:

- Do you have any form of heart disease?
- Do you have chest pain, or heaviness or other unusual sensations in your chest or neck?
- Have you ever had a heart attack?
- Have you ever had any surgery on your heart?
- Do you have any risk factors for heart disease, such as elevated cholesterol, obesity, a family history of heart disease, etc.?
- Do you have shortness of breath or have you ever had asthma?
- Do you smoke?
- Have you ever had liver disease?
- Have you ever had any kidney disease?
- Have you ever been told that you have circulatory problems? Do you think you have problems with your circulation?
- Are you or have you ever been depressed? Have you taken antidepressants?
- Have you ever been dependent on or addicted to any drugs, legal or illegal?
- How much alcohol do you drink?
- Are you pregnant? Planning to become pregnant? Breast-feeding?
- Have you ever had a bad reaction to any medicines?
- Have you ever had seizures or epilepsy?
- What medicines are you already taking?

- What vitamins, minerals, or other supplements are you taking?
- Have you ever had a bad reaction to any kind of medicine or supplement?

And that's just the beginning of the questions. But the conversation shouldn't end when you've been handed the prescription. Your doctor should carefully explain how to use the drug: how much to take, when and how, how to store the medicine, when to discard it, what potential warning signs to look for, and so forth.

If your doctor doesn't ask you the types of questions above, and many more, it may be time to get a new physician.

Chapter 11

———◄O►———

A Few Words on Sleep

- Do you go to bed later on Friday and Saturday nights because you don't have to get up and go to work the next day?
- Do you go to bed because the clock says it's bedtime, even if you're not tired?
- Do you stay in bed and try to force sleep when you are having trouble falling asleep?
- Do you nap during the day?
- Do you exercise less on days when you feel fatigued from lack of sleep?
- Do you eat, watch TV, work, talk on the phone, or read in bed?
- Do you try to catch up on missed sleep by sleeping late when you've got the chance?
- Do you drink alcoholic beverages or take sleeping medication to help you fall asleep?

- Do you drink caffeinated beverages after 3:00 P.M.?
- Do you smoke?

If you answered yes to any of these questions, you may be contributing to your migraines by interfering with normal, healthy sleep patterns. Surprisingly, not only can too little sleep trigger a migraine, *too much sleep can do the same!* Lack of sleep causes fatigue, irritability, and increased excitability of the nervous system, all of which can lower the "migraine threshold." Too much sleep alters the internal circadian rhythm: This has an effect on serotonin systems in the body, and serotonin plays a role in migraines. Whether too little or too much, the wrong amount of sleep can lead to trouble.

TOO MUCH SLEEP

Too much sleep is an easy problem to solve, once you know how much is too much. You can begin by eliminating all napping and keeping a sleep diary. Go to bed at the same time every night and set your alarm for your usual wake-up time. Then make sure you don't hit the snooze button and go back for a few more winks! Make a note in your diary of the amount of time you slept. If you wake up with a migraine, or develop one shortly after waking, adjust your sleeping time by either going to bed an hour later or getting up an hour earlier. Continue to experiment with your sleeping schedule, but don't cut back to less than six hours of sleep per night: That's the minimum that most people need to feel refreshed and ready to take on the day.

TOO LITTLE SLEEP

Lack of sleep is a far more common problem, and for migraineurs it can become part of a vicious circle that seems almost impossible to break. The migraine pain makes it hard to fall asleep and the lack of sleep helps perpetuate the migraine. Or too little sleep actually brings on the migraine, which then makes it even harder to doze off. Either way, problems falling asleep and staying asleep (collectively known as *insomnia*) often plague those with migraines and make everything worse.

Amber, a twenty-six-year-old marketing executive, is a typical example of a migraineur with sleep problems. "It's really unfair," she said. "When I get a migraine, I really need to be able to crawl into my bed, turn the lights out, and just sleep it off. And that's exactly when I can't sleep, because of the pain. I start feeling really anxious, even angry, because I *have* to get some sleep—I can actually feel my heart racing. It's the most frustrating experience. And that seems to make falling asleep even more impossible."

Amber is right—the more frustrated, angry, or anxious you feel about falling asleep, the less likely you are to accomplish your goal. And should insomnia continue night after night, stress, exhaustion, irritability, anxiety, and depression—not to mention migraines—can literally take over your life. Productivity, coping skills, moods, work life, and family life can all take a real nosedive due to the lack of sleep and the resultant migraines. So it's clear: You *must* get adequate rest and sleep to lower your stress levels, maintain your physical and mental health, and ward off migraines. Luckily, both insomnia and the plain old lack of sleep are often due to poor habits, and habits can be changed! Read through the suggestions below and find out how to make constructive changes in your sleep habits.

GO TO BED AND GET UP AT THE
SAME TIME EVERY DAY

If you have no trouble falling asleep or staying asleep, then getting enough sleep is just a matter of "working it into your schedule." Most people are sleep-deficient because they don't plan well enough—or don't have the discipline necessary to follow that plan. Jennifer, a nineteen-year-old college student, found that partying until 2:00 A.M. and pulling occasional all-nighter study sessions set her up for some major bouts of migraine headaches that sometimes lasted for days. But once she made it a point to go to bed at midnight and get up at 8:00 A.M.—no matter what day it was—her migraines virtually disappeared.

If you *do* have trouble falling or staying asleep, then it's even more important that you set up a firm sleep schedule. Susan, a forty-five-year-old paralegal and divorced mother of two, complained that she couldn't fall asleep at night and the lack of sleep was making her migraines worse. But after I interviewed her extensively about her lifestyle, it wasn't hard to figure out why. For one thing, she was beginning her workweek with a sleep deficit from which she never recovered. For example, at 10:00 P.M. on a Sunday night, Susan is just starting to get things organized for the week ahead. She needs to make and freeze sandwiches for the kids, wash her hair, give herself a manicure, and pack her bag for work. There's no way she'll get in bed before midnight—and she's got to get up at 6:30! If she had been more organized, she could have started making the kids' sandwiches right after dinner, then washed her hair and been ready to do her manicure by 9:00 P.M. That would leave her plenty of time to relax before turning in for the night.

Susan's got another bad habit: sleeping in on the weekends. After racing around all week on six-and-a-half, maybe seven hours of sleep per night, Saturday morning seems like heaven to her. The kids are with Susan's ex, so she's able to luxuriate in a nice long sleep that lasts until about 11:00 A.M. This is bad for two reasons: First, she wakes up with a migraine, which ruins the rest of her day. Second, her body "believes" that 11:00 A.M., her wake-up time, is really 6:30 A.M. (her usual wake-up time). It goes through the day completely out of sync with the actual time. When 11:00 P.M. rolls around, is her body going to be ready to go to sleep? Heck no—it thinks the night is still young! And if Susan goes out dancing, comes home at 2:00 A.M., then sleeps until 11:00 A.M. again, the pattern will be reinforced. She'll have terrible trouble falling asleep on Sunday night, even though that 6:30 A.M. wake-up call will be awaiting her on Monday.

You can see why it's so important to go to bed at the same time every single night, even on the weekends. You want to train your body to be ready for sleep soon after your head hits the pillow—and that will be difficult if your head is hitting the pillow at 11:00 P.M. some nights and 2:00 A.M. others. Your body has a rhythm to it; it works in a cyclical manner. Respect those cycles and use them to your benefit.

CREATE AN ENVIRONMENT THAT'S CONDUCIVE TO SLEEP

Even a good sleeper can have trouble falling and staying asleep in a bed that's not comfortable or a bedroom that's too hot, too cold, too bright, or too noisy. If you've got trouble sleeping, look first to your environment to make sure it's not the cause.

- *Keep it dark.* Do you have a streetlight that shines through your window? Does the morning sun wake you up too early? Does bright sunlight streaming through your window give you a morning migraine? If you answered yes to any of these questions, run, don't walk, to your nearest home furnishing store and invest in a set of heavy drapes—or a blackout shade, if allergies plague you. If you don't want to spend a lot of money, or if your partner likes a sunny bedroom, consider buying an eyeshade instead.

- *Keep it quiet.* Can you hear the sounds of traffic from your bedroom? Does your neighbor's dog bark incessantly through the night? Do dripping faucets, creaking foundations, argumentative neighbors, or snoring bed partners (either human, animal, or both!) keep you awake at night? Noise is a real bugaboo for most insomniacs, whose fragile sleep won't tolerate much in the way of intrusions. You can solve the problem by adding more noise—a background noise that can cover up the intermittent bursts of sound in your environment. An air conditioner, a fan, or a white noise machine can do the trick, providing a steady hum that helps the brain relax and settle into sleep.

- *Keep it cool.* A bedroom that is too warm can interfere with sleep because the body must drop to a certain temperature before it can enter into sleep. If your body temperature doesn't decrease or decreases slowly, you'll have trouble falling asleep and staying asleep. Deep sleep will be reduced, and middle-of-the-night awakenings increased. That's why people generally get less sleep during the hot nights of summer, but sleep great during the cool nights of fall and winter. To maximize the length and quality of your sleep, keep your bedroom cool, but use enough warm blankets to stay comfortable. (If you're too cold, you won't sleep well either!) Turn down the heat before you go to bed on cool nights, keeping the temperature between 55 and 65 degrees. On warm nights, use an air conditioner, open a window (if it's quiet outside), or turn on a fan, if necessary, to create your own "good sleeping weather."

- *Keep it comfortable.* If your mattress is too soft, too hard, too lumpy, or has a well in the middle that you roll into regularly, you can bet you're not sleeping as well as you could. Invest in a good-quality mattress—but be sure to test it before you buy. I have a friend who recently bought a new mattress and went for the extra-firm variety because everyone kept telling her, "Get something firm!" But the mattress turned out to be so rock-hard she felt like she was lying on cement! Don't take anybody else's word for it; buy what feels best to you. You may also want to get a good mattress cover that will allow the angles of your body to sink into it rather than run up against the mattress proper, which will be less resilient.

  Pillows are another sticking point for many would-be sleepers. Get one that supports your head and neck but doesn't prop your head up at an unnatural angle. (That puts a strain on your neck and can lead to neckaches and headaches.) Choosing the right pillow will be a very individual matter, since each person assumes his or her own unique sleeping positions. Get a pillow that will allow you to keep your neck and spine in a straight line while you sleep.

  Sleeping on your side is the position recommended by most health experts. Tuck a pillow under the side of your head to keep the spine straight, and another one between your knees so you won't have to twist your hips toward the mattress to support your legs. If you like to sleep on your back, get a cervical pillow (shaped like a cylinder) and put it underneath the back of your neck, so that your shoulders and the top of your head contact the mattress. Put another pillow beneath your knees, keeping them bent, which will take the strain off your back. If you like to sleep on your stomach, however, it's best to try to break the habit. Sleeping on your stomach causes your lower back to sway and strains the neck.

CONSIDER GOING IT ALONE

Although it doesn't sound very romantic, sleeping by yourself is one of the best ways to get a good night's sleep. Many people swear that sleeping with their partner makes them feel more relaxed and cozy, leading to improved sleep quality, but studies have shown just the opposite. Bed partners do much to interrupt the other's sleep—snoring, kicking, hogging the bed or the blankets, and observing differing sleeping schedules. Plus, every time your partner rolls over or jostles the bed, you wake up, whether you know it or not.

If you're having trouble falling or staying asleep, consider investing in a set of twin beds, or sleeping in another bedroom. That doesn't have to preclude romance. You can spend all the time you like snuggling in bed with your partner; just get up and go to another bed when it's time to sleep.

Restless Leg Can Lead to an Unrestful Night

Restless leg syndrome is a very common—and commonly underdiagnosed—condition that can cause headaches and many other unpleasant symptoms. Although it's a lifelong illness, many who have it consider it to be normal, because they've had it for so long.

The syndrome consists of very unpleasant, but not painful, sensations in the legs, or perhaps the entire body. These sensations become unbearable unless the affected part of the body is moved. In mild cases the syndrome strikes only at night, but severe cases can cause fidgeting all day long. Even in mild cases, however, people continue moving while they're asleep, and this prevents them from going into the deep, restful stages of sleep. Victims may wake up exhausted after eight hours of sleep because they never stopped moving. It's the bed partners who often draw attention to the syndrome, because it may ruin their sleep as well.

You should consult with your physician if you have or think you have restless leg syndrome, which is sometimes caused by iron deficiency and a nerve dysfunction. Several prescription drugs can be very helpful, including some used to treat Parkinson's disease and certain opioids. (They shouldn't cause addiction because they're usually taken only before going to sleep.)

USE THE BED FOR TWO THINGS ONLY

In Mary Norton's book *Bed-Knob and Broomstick*, three children are able to use their bed to fly to distant lands for fantastic adventures played out during the course of the night. Then, just as dawn is breaking, the children and their flying bed return to their bedroom, landing with a screech and a thump. I bring this up because it reminds me of the way many people use their beds. (Well, sort of!) That is, the bed is used for all sorts of things that have nothing to do with sleeping! Watching television and videos, eating entire meals, playing with the children and the pets, writing, doing office work, balancing the checkbook—you name it! If you can do it sitting down, it seems, people are doing it in bed.

But the unfortunate result of all of this bed-centered activity is that the bed is no longer associated with sleep alone. In your great-grandmother's day, people went to their bedrooms to dress and to sleep. Once they were awake, they went downstairs to huddle around the stove (most bedrooms weren't heated!), cook meals, or get ready to go out and plow the back forty. When they went to their bedrooms at night, the cue to sleep was very strong. (It helped that they went to bed about the same time every night, right about when the last coals were dying down.)

We, however, don't tend to see the bed and think "sleep." It's more like "a comfortable place to snuggle up and live." But you can retrain yourself so that the sight of your bed at night will automatically make you feel sleepy. You'll just have to stay out of the bedroom until it's time to sleep! Use your bed for two things only: sleep and sex. Everything else should be done in another room. Watch TV in the den, do your bills in your home office, eat in the dining room. Don't bring all of these complications into the bedroom.

GET SOME EXERCISE—EVERY DAY!

Studies have shown that people who have trouble sleeping tend to get less exercise than those who sleep normally. That's too bad, because regular exercise can help make it easier to fall asleep. It does so because the temperature of the body assumes a gradual rise and fall during the day, with the fall encouraging sleep onset. (Indeed, sleeping in a room that's too warm can inhibit this fall in body temperature, making sleep elusive. Think of tossing and turning on hot summer nights!) But exercise can help you fall asleep more easily by causing a significant rise in body temperature, followed by a drop that lasts for at least a few hours. So if you exercise between three and six hours before bedtime, you can play into this resulting drop in body temperature and get a little extra help falling asleep. Make sure you have a gap of at least three hours between your exercise session and bedtime, however. Otherwise your temperature may still be too high for the sleep cycle to begin.

Exercise can also help improve the quality of sleep. The brain naturally increases the amount of deep sleep you experience in response to the physical stress of exercise, so you should sleep soundly after you've had a good workout session.

EAT WITH CAUTION

Although warm milk and whole-grain crackers may help ease you into blissful sleep, there are a few things you *shouldn't* eat or drink within a few hours of bedtime:

- *Alcoholic beverages.* Although initially alcohol may relax you and make you feel sleepy, it actually suppresses deep sleep, making sleep lighter and more fragmented. And as it's metabolized during the night, alcohol interrupts sleep by producing mild withdrawal symptoms that cause more frequent awakenings and lighter sleep. It also suppresses dream sleep, which the body counteracts with intense dreams or nightmares during the second half of the night that can increase the number of awakenings. And when alcohol is used regularly as a way to fall asleep, it can become a crutch that might end in alcoholism. It's estimated that 10 percent of alcoholics get started this way.
- *Caffeinated foods and beverages.* You can forget that cup of hot cocoa before bed, or the chocolate-covered candy bar. Anything containing caffeine (coffee, tea, chocolate, cocoa, soft drinks, etc.) can stimulate you, and should be avoided after 6:00 P.M. If you're particularly sensitive to caffeine, make 3:00 P.M. your deadline or cut it out of your diet completely.

- *Heavy meals.* The digestive system naturally slows down as the night wears on, so digesting a heavy meal (say, one eaten after about 8:00 P.M.) will be more difficult. The resulting indigestion, or just the flurry of bodily activity, may make sleep more elusive. Eat your meal earlier, or if you must eat late, eat light. It's a good idea to drink fluid sparingly after 8:00 P.M. also, to reduce middle-of-the-night bathroom trips.

- *High-sugar foods.* Sugary foods and foods high in refined carbohydrates (cookies, cake, candy, etc.) increase blood sugar levels and give the body extra energy right when it doesn't need it. Eat a light snack containing complex carbohydrates (whole-grain bread, crackers, bagels, etc.) instead.

- *Gassy foods.* Foods that cause intestinal gas, indigestion, or heartburn (for instance, beans, cucumbers, spicy foods, high-fat foods, garlic, onions, etc.) can wreak havoc on your digestive system right when you don't need the distraction. Eat these foods much earlier in the day.

- *High-protein foods.* Foods high in protein can interfere with the synthesis of serotonin, the feel-good hormone that helps us fall asleep. Avoid eggs, meat, poultry, fish, cheese, and nuts for at least two hours before bedtime.

- *Foods containing MSG.* MSG (monosodium glutamate) acts as a stimulant in some people and should be avoided before bedtime (if not always).

WATCH YOUR DRUG CONSUMPTION

Sleeping Medications

All too often, a person with frequent or chronic sleeping problems finds herself trapped in a dependency on prescription sleeping pills. At first, sleeping medications may seem a godsend for the frustrated, anxious insomniac who wonders how she'll make it through the day without adequate sleep. And initially, the little pills usually *do* help reduce the amount of time it takes to fall asleep, as well as the number of nighttime awakenings. But over time, sleeping pills tend to become less and less effective, and a person requires more and more medication to achieve the same results. Or the person may also develop a psychological dependence, believing that she can't fall asleep without the drugs, even though no physical dependence exists. Either way, the upshot is that she finds herself unable to fall asleep without the drugs; she's addicted.

Other side effects include "morning-after" impairment in thinking and coordination, drowsiness, lethargy, dizziness, blurred vision, high blood pressure, anxiety, and digestive upsets. On the psychological front, the person may suffer from a lowered self-esteem, increased anxiety levels, and a feeling of being out of control. Where once she just had trouble falling asleep, now she's facing addiction. And her sleep problem may be even worse.

Because of their wide range of potentially dangerous side effects, sleeping medications should be used for a short time only (no more than two or three weeks) if they're used at all. Keep in mind that they don't attack the root cause of the insomnia; they only mask the symptoms. They do nothing to train your brain to fall asleep naturally or point the way toward any real solution, and they can actually disturb both deep sleep and REM sleep.

Sleeping pills may be useful on occasion: say, when you're experiencing jet lag or the night before an important event. But they should be taken in the smallest dose possible and should never be used on consecutive nights. If you've had two bad nights and are experiencing a third, take a small dose. But always observe the good sleep habits outlined in this chapter as your first-line defense against insomnia, relying on medications only when absolutely necessary.

There is no hard evidence supporting the effectiveness of over-the-counter medications (such as Nytol, Sominex, Unisom, Tylenol PM, Excedrin P.M., etc.), and some people have reported that their use caused daytime drowsiness, increased anxiety, and psychological dependence. As with prescription sleeping aids, avoid anything other than occasional use.

Other Medications That Cause Insomnia

An amazing number of prescriptions and over-the-counter drugs can short-circuit the amount and quality of your sleep. Some act as stimulants; others interfere with dream sleep or deep sleep; still others can ruin your sleep via the effects of their withdrawal. Consult with your physician about changing prescriptions if your medication is adversely affecting your sleep, or ask your pharmacist for recommendations if an over-the-counter drug is doing the same. Sometimes just changing brands or taking your dose earlier in the day may be all you need.

FYI, the most common over-the-counter and prescription drugs that can interfere with sleep include the following:

- Certain antidepressants (such as Prozac)
- Asthma medications
- Beta-blockers and certain other high blood pressure medications
- Over-the-counter drugs that contain caffeine, including pain relievers (such as Anacin, Excedrin Extra-Strength, Vanquish, Bromo-Seltzer, Cope, and Midol); diet pills (Dexatrim); diuretics (Aqua-Ban); and stimulants (NoDoz, Vivarin)

- Nasal decongestants that contain stimulants
- Parkinson's disease medications
- Prescription analgesics that contain caffeine (such as Cafergot, Damason-P, Darvon Compound-65, Esgic, Fioricet, Fiorinal, Norgesic, Norgesic Forte)
- Steroids
- Thyroid medication

Smoking

Smoking can also bring about a decrease in deep sleep and more frequent nighttime awakenings. That's because of the stimulating effects of nicotine and the withdrawal symptoms that can show themselves after just a few nonsmoking hours (like right in the middle of the night!). If you smoke at or near bedtime or upon awakening during the night, you're just exacerbating the problem. Do whatever it takes to quit smoking. You'll sleep better, and probably experience fewer migraines in the bargain.

WIND DOWN BEFORE BEDTIME

It's also important to take some time to relax before you go to bed. Racing around the house doing last-minute chores then falling into bed exhausted is a great way to ensure you'll be lying there counting sheep for the next couple of hours. You wouldn't ride a racehorse at top speed around the track, then gallop up to the stable door and just shut him in for the night. You'd walk him around the track at a leisurely pace, then smooth him down and make other preparations for the night. Treat yourself in the same general way. Spend at least an hour before bedtime doing quiet, relaxing things in preparation for sleep. Take a nice warm bath. Listen to soft music; do some yoga or other stretches; meditate. Drink some herbal tea (chamomile or valerian). Eat a light carbohydrate snack or drink a cup of warm milk. (Carbohydrates and milk encourage the production of the hormone serotonin, which helps induce sleep.) Anything to downshift your body's machinery from high gear to idle.

DON'T GO TO BED UNTIL YOU'RE SLEEPY

Even though I've said that you need to stick to a sleep schedule, you also need to respect what's going on in your body. The body will not be forced; it has a will of its own. The most important thing about a sleep schedule is getting up at the same time every day. (Here you *can* force it!) But wait until your body tells you it's sleepy before getting into bed. If you're getting up at the same time every day, the urge to go to sleep at a particular time should come up naturally. If it's not happening at your designated bedtime, maybe you need less sleep than you think. So stay up—do some light reading, watch a little television, fold laundry, or do some other easy, monotonous chore. Do *not* lie down, however. Save that for when you get into bed. The idea is to make your bed a place where you want to go, not a place to fear or dread.

IF YOU CAN'T FALL ASLEEP, GET UP!

When you finally feel sleepy, go to bed. Relax and try not to go over the events of the day or do any heavy thinking. If, after about thirty minutes, you still haven't fallen asleep, get up. This may be hard to do—it's cold, you feel like you've failed, and so on—but it's absolutely necessary. You don't want to toss and turn and begin to associate bed with a lack of sleep.

Go back to reading or doing a monotonous chore and don't lie down. Stay up for at least thirty minutes. When you feel sleepy, go back to bed. Repeat this sequence as many times as necessary until you fall asleep. Eventually your mind should associate sleep with your bed and help you fall asleep easily and naturally.

DON'T TRY TO FORCE IT

One of the worse things you can do is to get in bed and say to yourself, "Okay, now I've *got* to fall asleep!" Sleep is one of those elusive things. It seems like the more you chase after it, the farther away it gets. In a way, you have to pretend you don't really care, and then it will come slinking around like a spurned lover. But if you get upset or angry or anxious because you're not falling asleep fast enough—forget it! You'll be in the worst frame of mind for falling asleep. Relax, you probably need less sleep than you think. Researchers have found that daytime performance doesn't usually suffer as long as you get about five and a half hours of core sleep (deep sleep), and if you don't get it one night, your body will do whatever it can to get it the next night.

Chapter 12

◄○►

A Note on Women and Migraines

*I*t seems unfair, doesn't it, that a full 70 percent of migraine sufferers are women! And yet if you look at boys and girls under the age of eleven or so, you'll find that the sexes have roughly the same incidence of headache. Ditto men and women past the age of fifty-five. The big increase in migraines in women occurs during the childbearing years. Many women experience their first migraine either at menarche, once they begin using birth control pills, while they're pregnant, or during the postpartum period. Add the fact that 70 percent of women experience their worst headaches within a few days of the onset of their monthly periods and a picture begins to form: Migraines are often connected to female hormone levels. Indeed, researchers studying the effects of the rise and fall of hormone levels during the normal course of the menstrual cycle have found that there are certain times when a woman is much more likely to develop a migraine, for example at ovulation or during the week before menses. Unfortunately, these are also the times when a migraine may be more resistant to standard medications.

PMS

Experts estimate that between 30 and 60 percent of menstruating women (up to 40 million Americans!) suffer from premenstrual syndrome (PMS), a group of symptoms that occurs prior to menstruation, and often includes headaches (sometimes called "menstrual migraines"). Besides headaches, typical symptoms of PMS include mood swings, bloating, irritability, depression, backaches, skin disorders, breast tenderness, binge eating, and weight gain. Since the origins of PMS and menstrual migraines appear to be the same (hormonal), let's take a look at what goes on during the menstrual cycle to find out what might be causing so much misery.

THE RISE AND FALL OF THE HORMONES

The menstrual cycle is governed by two hormones, estrogen and progesterone, each of which rises and falls independently of the other. The entire menstrual cycle takes approximately four weeks (28 days), with the first day of menstruation deemed Day 1 of the cycle. From Day 1 through Day 14, the uterus prepares itself to receive a fertilized egg, and at the beginning of this phase both estrogen and progesterone levels are at their lowest. On subsequent days, estrogen levels gradually rise, reaching a peak just before ovulation, which occurs about Day 14. Typically, the incidence of menstrual migraines is low during this first half of the cycle.

At ovulation (or just slightly before), estrogen levels begin to decline somewhat, and, although they don't fall to their original Day 1 level, they continue to decline for a few days before beginning another rise. Levels reach their second peak in the cycle at around Day 23 (or five days before menstruation). Meanwhile, progesterone levels, which begin to rise immediately after ovulation, also reach their peak around Day 23. Then, during the next five days, the levels of both hormones plummet, triggering the breakdown of the endometrium (lining of the uterus) and the onset of menses, which occurs on Day 1 of the new cycle.

Most likely, it's the precipitous drop in hormone levels from Day 23 to Day 28 that brings on PMS and menstrual migraines. To make matters worse, the body produces greater amounts of a hormone called *prostaglandin* in response to these hormonal swings, and prostaglandin increases sensitivity to pain. Many women who experience menstrual migraines are symptom-free during the first two weeks of the menstrual cycle, then develop headaches sometime during the two-week period before menstruation begins. The drop in estrogen associated with ovulation (Day 14) triggers migraines in a few women, but most often these headaches occur during the week or so before the onset of menstruation, as estrogen and progesterone levels begin their rapid decline. Hormone fluctuations are also the most likely cause of migraines during pregnancy. During the first trimester, when estrogen levels change drastically, migraines can be frequent, although they usually decrease or disappear altogether during the second and third trimesters, when hormone levels stabilize.

Of course, not every woman gets a migraine during the week before her period, while pregnant, or after menopause. But for those who do, the cause is probably one or more of the following:

- a sudden drop in hormone levels
- estrogen levels that are too low
- estrogen levels that are too high
- progesterone levels that are too low

Most of the time, it's the sudden drop in hormone levels that triggers migraines, although for some, the absolute level may be the problem.

TOO LITTLE OR TOO MUCH?

Low levels of estrogen clearly affect the serotonin receptors, setting the stage for the onset of many of the symptoms of PMS, including pain, irritability, depression, hot flashes, night sweats, vaginal dryness, and—no surprise—migraines. (Remember that changes in serotonin can lead to the dilation of the blood vessels that is the hallmark of these headaches.)

Lots of things can contribute to decreased estrogen levels, including:

- menopause
- cigarette smoking
- too little body fat
- stress
- too much exercise
- nutritional deficiencies

But estrogen levels that are too high can also cause PMS and migraine headaches. Fatigue, insomnia, anxiety, depression, low blood sugar, emotional hypersensitivity, and blood platelet clumping are all brought about by an excess of estrogen, and each of these symptoms increases the likelihood of migraines.

High levels of estrogen also cause the retention of both fluid and salt (think of premenstrual bloating, breast tenderness, and weight gain), and fluid retention itself can be an indirect cause of migraines. In addition, excess estrogen causes magnesium deficiency and a reduced supply of oxygen to the cells, both potent headache triggers.

Estrogen excess can be the result of one or more of the following:

- birth control pills
- estrogen-only hormone replacement therapy
- excess body fat (fatty tissue produces estrogen)
- stress
- impaired liver function
- poor diet

We also live in an "estrogen-laden society," which can drive up our levels of this hormone through our exposure to:

- meats
- pesticides
- furnishings
- soaps
- plastics
- industrial wastes

And, oddly enough, you can find yourself suffering from the symptoms of estrogen excess even if your estrogen levels are *low,* as long as your progesterone levels also happen to be low. That's because progesterone counterbalances the effects of estrogen— sort of like yin and yang. If progesterone is scarce, the system is thrown out of whack and even small amounts of estrogen can bring about a condition known as *estrogen dominance.* This explains why the symptoms of estrogen excess can occur during the premenstrual period when estrogen levels are actually in decline: Progesterone levels are also in decline, and they may fall low enough to cause estrogen dominance.

PROGESTERONE TO THE RESCUE

In a healthy body, progesterone acts in opposition to estrogen. For example, estrogen increases the proliferation of body fat, while progesterone helps break down that fat for use as energy. Estrogen increases fluid retention, while progesterone has a natural diuretic action. Estrogen slows the sex drive; progesterone restores it.

Progesterone has many and varied effects on the body and the mind, including some that may help prevent the symptoms of PMS and migraines:

- natural antidepressant action
- blood sugar stabilization
- stabilization of cell oxygen levels
- natural diuretic action
- restoration of vascular tone
- anti-inflammatory effects
- normalization of sleep patterns

Unfortunately, in many people estrogen levels are either unnaturally high or progesterone levels are extremely low (seen in those who don't ovulate or who are postmenopausal), so the anti-PMS effects provided by naturally produced progesterone may not be evident. In these cases, progesterone replacement may be necessary. Many women have found relief from their PMS symptoms and/or menstrual migraines through the use of a natural progesterone cream or oral progesterone. Consult your physician if you think this might help you.

MENOPAUSE, ORAL CONTRACEPTIVES, AND MIGRAINES

Fortunately, many women stop having migraines after menopause, and men also tend to have fewer migraines once they reach their fifties. For both sexes, the presumed cause of this decline in migraines is the age-related reduction in the number of serotonin receptors.

In some women, however, the headaches worsen during the transition period, during the onset of menopause when hormones are fluctuating. Hormone replacement therapy or, early in menopause, an oral contraceptive can sometimes relieve these wild fluctuations. I usually advise using an estrogen and progesterone skin patch.

While about 25 percent of women migraineurs find migraine relief through the use of oral contraceptives, another 25 percent find that birth control pills actually bring on migraines or make them worse, while 50 percent are not affected at all. A word of caution: Both migraines and the pill cause a very small increase in the risk of stroke. This does not mean that women with migraines should never take the pill, but it does mean that if you have additional risk factors for stroke, you should either try to eliminate these factors or stop taking oral contraceptives. Additional risk factors include smoking, high cholesterol, hypertension, and Syndrome X.[1]

---

[1] To learn about Syndrome X, read *Syndrome X: Overcoming the Silent Killer Than Can Give You A Heart Attack,* by Gerald Reaven, M.D. (New York: Simon & Schuster, 2000).

WHAT ABOUT MAGNESIUM, B₂, AND FEVERFEW?

One of the many detrimental effects of estrogen excess is magnesium deficiency. Studies have shown that women generally tend to have reduced magnesium levels during the premenstrual phase, and those with PMS may have even lower magnesium levels than normal women. Low magnesium also appears to be responsible for premenstrual migraines and is seen routinely in those who use oral contraceptives or estrogen-only hormone replacement therapy. Magnesium deficiency, as mentioned earlier, results in blood vessel constriction and the release of substance P, which brings on inflammation and pain. Taking a magnesium supplement of 300–400 mg per day (a recommended part of the "triple therapy") may reduce the incidence of menstrual migraines, while simultaneously easing other premenstrual symptoms, including cramps, depression, and water retention.

In many of those who take birth control pills, riboflavin levels are quite low. High levels of estrogen as well as too much stress also tend to deplete the B vitamins in general. My recommendations for riboflavin as part of the triple therapy should be of help in this area.

Feverfew has been found to be effective in quelling premenstrual headaches, reducing inflammation, and relieving menstrual cramps, as well as reducing the blood vessel spasms that bring on menstrual migraines. Those who are pregnant should avoid feverfew, however, since we are still unsure of the effect of herbal remedies on the fetus.

As you can see, the triple therapy can deliver a triple whammy to some painful problems that are especially vexing to women. Those who have menstrual migraines or PMS or those who take the birth control pill all stand to benefit from this safe, natural approach.

Chapter 13

———◀O▶———

Questions and Answers about the Triple Therapy

What's the extent of the migraine problem in this country?

It's a tremendous problem. Over 25 million Americans suffer from the excruciating headaches, as well as the nausea and other symptoms of the syndrome. We spend more than $20 billion a year looking for relief from migraines.

What causes migraines?

Although we have several good theories, we can't say exactly what happens in the brain to trigger a migraine. It may have to do with disturbances of serotonin in the brain, irritation of certain nerves, or another problem. For whatever reason, the blood vessels in the brain contract then dilate inappropriately, setting the migraine in motion.

What's the difference between migraines and other headaches?

There are many types of headaches, including migraines, tension headaches, cluster headaches, and exertion headaches.

Usually a physician can give you the diagnosis of a migraine headache, which typically produces pain that grips one side of your head, is moderate to severe, and lasts anywhere from a couple hours to days. Any headache that impairs normal functioning is most likely a migraine.

Oddly enough, despite the fact that migraines can produce terrible pain and other symptoms, a fair number of sufferers go undiagnosed and do not receive proper treatment.

Are migraines limited to the head?

Migraines are much more than pain in the head: They're a full-body syndrome complete with nausea, intolerance of light and sound, sweating, double vision, bright spots before the eyes, numbness and tingling in the face and hands, confused thinking, slurred speech, weakness of the limbs, diarrhea, chills, sometimes auras, and other symptoms.

Who is most likely to get migraines?

Women are the syndrome's favorite targets: 70 percent of migraineurs are female. Although migraines can strike people of any age, from early childhood to the golden years, adolescents and young adults are most likely to suffer.

Why do women suffer more than men?

We don't really know. Changing levels of hormones during a woman's monthly cycle may trigger the headaches. It's also possible that the increasing stress many women face, as they try to work and raise families, is a contributing factor.

What are "classic" and "common" migraines?

"Classic" and "common" are old terms. Today we call the classic type a migraine with aura, while the common type is known as a migraine without aura.

There are other types of migraines, including the menstrual migraine, basilar migraine, hemiplegic migraine, ophthalmo-plegic migraine, and retinal migraine.

Are women immune to migraines while they're pregnant?

Not necessarily. For about 25 percent of pregnant women, pregnancy has no effect on their migraines. For many, the migraines may get better, and for some, they may get worse.

Do migraines in women disappear after menopause?

Sometimes. Some women are lucky enough to say good-bye to their migraines as they move through menopause. But for others, the problem can grow worse.

How about kids? Do they get migraines?

Unfortunately, yes. The migraines suffered by youngsters may be very similar to those that strike adults or very different. Children might have pain on both sides of the head, rather than only one. And the pain may be relatively brief, perhaps lasting only a few hours or less. In addition to the pain, the youngsters may suffer from nausea, the "blahs," sensitivity to light, sound, and strong odors, and other symptoms.

What are the phases of a migraine?

A migraine may begin with the *prodrome*, complete with sensitivity to light, noise, touch, and smell; there may also be mood changes, memory problems, or other disturbances. Then comes the *aura*, the visual disturbance that heralds migraines in perhaps 15 percent of sufferers. Next is the headache itself, often accompanied by nausea, weakness, dizziness, and other prob-lems, lasting for hours or days. The headache fades away during the *resolution* period; then you enter into the *postdrome*, the "after-event" phase in which you feel tired and miserable for up to a day.

Not every migraine follows this set pattern, of course.

What are migraine triggers?

These are the things, mind-sets, or situations that seem to bring on migraines. It's felt that migraineurs have "headaches waiting to happen," but that the headaches won't begin until set off by the trigger. Triggers are very individual: What turns your head into "a nuclear battleground" may have absolutely no effect on another migraineur.

What are some common triggers?

Cheese, bacon, nuts, avocados, chocolate, yeast, spices, hot dogs, corn, or anything fermented, as well as red wine, beer, or beverages and other edibles containing caffeine are common triggers. So are stress, fatigue, bright lights, strong odors, certain medications, perfumes or other odors, air pollution, hormonal changes, skipping meals, the weather, seasonal changes, and altitude.

Do triggers always set off migraines?

Not all of them, not always. Some people can get away with a little exposure to a trigger, especially if everything else is going well. For example, they may be able to eat one orange with no problem, but a headache will develop if they consume two. Or, if they're under a lot of stress, just one orange may be all it takes to trigger a migraine. But sometimes migraines strike without obvious triggers.

Are migraines genetic?

The latest research suggests that most people with migraine headaches have minor genetic abnormalities that make them more susceptible to migraines. But remember, simply having "migraine genes" is not enough: You must also be exposed to your trigger.

Why don't standard medicines work?

They do work, to a certain extent. For many people, standard medicines such as Imitrex, Maxalt, and Cafergot do a good job of relieving migraines in progress—but they don't prevent future ones from striking. Neither do they make "the next one" any gentler or shorter. But some people, unfortunately, don't respond well to these or similar medicines. They must make their way to the doctor's office or an emergency room where they can receive an injection of more potent medicines. And all medicines have side effects, sometimes very serious ones.

What is the "triple therapy"?

The triple therapy is an all-natural, very safe and effective method of preventing migraines. The three ingredients in the therapy are the mineral magnesium, the vitamin riboflavin (vitamin B_2), and the herb feverfew. The dosages are 300–400 mg of magnesium, 400 mg of riboflavin, and 100 mg of feverfew per day. Break your total dosage in half, and take it in two doses per day, with meals. You can purchase the three ingredients individually, or in a "combination" pill such as MigraHealth™ (available in drug stores and independent pharmacies nationwide).

How does magnesium help relieve migraines?

A large number of migraineurs have low levels of a particular form of magnesium known as serum ionized magnesium. Replacing what's missing relieves migraines in progress, and can prevent future ones as well.

Magnesium does many of the same good things that successful migraine drugs do. For example, this mineral helps keep the blood vessels in the brain properly toned and open, allowing the blood to flow freely. It also prevents the arteries from going into sudden spasm, and helps keep nerve cell membranes stable, among other things. In these ways, magnesium acts as a "medicine" for migraines. The mineral can also help make other migraine drugs more effective.

How does riboflavin help with migraines?

I must confess that we don't really know. We do know that the vitamin is involved in energy generation in each cell of the body, and we can point to the studies that show that taking the vitamin can significantly reduce the number of migraines that strike.

What's the link between feverfew and migraine relief?

We don't really know. The best theory is that the sesquiterpene lactones and other ingredients in the herb help regulate brain chemistry and quell the inflammation process.

Is the "triple therapy" real science, or just another overhyped cure-of-the-month that will quickly disappear?

The triple therapy is based on solid scientific evidence, plus experience with hundreds of patients at my New York Headache Center and elsewhere. The research has been conducted by various teams of scientists in this country and abroad, and presented in prestigious journals such as *Headache* and *Neurology.* A fair number of the studies have been double-blind and placebo-controlled, which means they're scientifically rigorous and valid.

Is the triple therapy by itself enough?

For many people, the triple therapy is all it takes to make

migraines nothing more than an occasional problem. Some, in fact, do quite well on just one or two of the three ingredients. Others need all three, or the full Banishing Migraines Program (see chapter 5). And many people obtain significant relief from the triple therapy, but still need other nonpharmacological and drug therapies.

What's the full Banishing Migraines Program?

It's a complete program for combating migraines. It touches all the bases, so even if a lack of magnesium or riboflavin isn't your problem, and even if feverfew isn't the cure for you, you can still benefit from the full program. Here are the seven steps.

1. Get a proper diagnosis from a medical doctor. Make sure that you're really suffering from migraines.
2. Use the triple therapy to significantly reduce or eliminate your migraines.
3. Identify and avoid your migraine triggers.
4. Eat to avoid migraines.
5. Take the edge off. Reduce the stress that may be lowering your threshold to migraines or making your life more miserable than it has to be after the headaches strike.
6. Walk it off. Exercise is a great way to strengthen your overall health and to raise the pain threshold by reducing stress.
7. Use medicines as necessary. There's no such thing as a perfect program. It takes a while for the triple therapy to kick in, and even then you may still suffer from occasional migraines. Standard medicine can help you deal with the headaches that do strike.

Will the triple therapy help with other problems besides migraines?

Undoubtedly. One part of the therapy has helped patients suffering from cluster headaches. And the magnesium in the therapy is also used to help certain people suffering from heart disease, asthma, PMS, and other problems.

What are cluster headaches?

Cluster headaches are groups or series of headaches that can be so painful they've been dubbed "suicide headaches." They come in groups, one or several per day over many days, weeks, or months, and typically last between 30 and 90 minutes. The pain usually starts mildly in the upper half of one side of your face, and quickly escalates, apparently centering itself right behind the eye on the affected side of your face. That eye becomes teary, possibly bloodshot, and droopy, while the nostril on the pained side of your face runs or stuffs up. The pain is so intense that you may feel like pacing, rocking back and forth, or even hitting your head rather than lying still.

Men between the ages of twenty and forty are the primary targets of cluster headaches.

What are tension headaches?

These are the run-of-the-mill headaches we may suffer after a trying experience. Tension headaches usually produce mild to moderate, steady pain that most describe as a dull ache. The pain comes on gradually, and spreads over both sides of your head. Your neck and shoulder muscles may be tense, but you don't feel nauseous, have no visual disturbances, and are not unusually sensitive to light, movement, or sound (as you would be with a migraine). Ninety percent of the headaches we suffer from are tension headaches, and they usually respond well to over-the-counter pain remedies.

What are exertion headaches?

They are headaches triggered by physical activity such as laughing, exercising, coughing, or engaging in sex. They can be painful but are not usually dangerous. Still, it's best to have them checked out, because they may be signaling a stroke or some other serious problem.

What are organic headaches?

These are headaches caused by other problems, such as a brain tumor or a head injury. Only a tiny percentage of headaches are organic, but they can herald very serious trouble, so you should be checked out right away if you notice any of these signs:

- The pain is new; that is, you haven't had this type of headache before.
- The pain is coupled with a fever, stiff neck, or other unusual symptoms.
- When the pain strikes, or soon after, you're confused, have difficulty moving or speaking, and feel very tired or faint.
- The pain begins after you've had a head injury.
- The pain gets worse with each new headache, or headaches become more and more frequent.

Why should I keep a headache diary?

One of the keys to combating migraines is to identify the triggers and assess the results of treatment, including the triple therapy. The diary is very important, for many people don't remember exactly how many headaches they had before and after the treatment started. And identifying triggers can be a very complex process, so it helps to know what you've eaten, where you've been, what you've been doing, how you are feeling, and what you may have been exposed to before your migraines strike.

One last question: Can I jump right into the triple therapy?

No. Speak to your physician first. Be sure to tell him or her what you want to do, and review all the elements of the program together.

Appendix—
Some Additional Studies

My colleagues and I were encouraged by the results of our first study with magnesium, which showed that low levels of serum ionized magnesium (IMg^{2+}), rather than total magnesium, were linked to migraine headaches in many people. We attempted to duplicate and expand the findings with a larger group of patients. For this study, we measured the amount of biologically active, ionized magnesium in the serum of two hundred consecutive patients at my New York Headache Center.[1] We then carefully scrutinized the results of the blood tests in the seventy-four patients who were actually having headaches when we drew the blood. Of those, thirty-two had acute migraine without aura, twenty-one had chronic daily headache of the migrainous type, twelve had chronic daily tension-type headache, and nine had acute tension headache.

The results were clear: The levels of biologically active, ion-

---

[1] Mauskop A, Altura BT, Cracco RQ, Altura BM. "Serum ionized magnesium levels in patients with tension-type headaches." In *Tension-type Headache: Classification, Mechanisms, and Treatment.* Olesen J and Schoenen J, eds. NY: Raven Press, 1993, pp 137–140.

ized magnesium in the serum were significantly lower in many of the people suffering from acute migraines, as well as in a fair number of those with chronic daily migrainous headaches and chronic daily tension-type headaches. Here are the breakdowns:

Type of headache	% with low IMg^{2+}
Acute migraine	41%
Chronic daily migrainous	24%
Chronic daily tension	33%
Acute tension	8%

Not only did we show that people in the throes of a headache had less biologically active, ionized magnesium in their serum, but all groups had a "significantly elevated $ICa^{2+}:IMg^{2+}$." In other words, they had too much serum ionized calcium compared to serum ionized magnesium. And too much calcium can produce problems similar to those seen with too little magnesium.

These findings supported the idea that some patients with migraine and other types of headaches may be lacking the vitally important serum ionized magnesium, possibly because their bodies have difficulty handling the mineral.

MAGNESIUM CAN MAKE STANDARD MEDICINE MORE EFFECTIVE

After several years of study, it was clear that measuring levels of magnesium could help us identify who was most likely to suffer migraines, and that supplemental magnesium could relieve and/or prevent attacks. Then we found that the mineral could do more: It could also potentiate standard medications.

Thirty to 35 percent of those with migraines do not respond to sumatriptan, an often-prescribed drug. Could there be a link between the lack of response and a lack of magnesium in the body? In 1998, a group of researchers tested this idea and presented their findings to their colleagues.[2]

Twenty migraineurs who reported no response to sumatriptan, or only a poor response, sought out help at a headache clinic. Blood tests showed that they had low levels of magnesium. Twelve of the twenty were then given ten IV infusions of magnesium (1 gm $MgSO_4$) over the next two weeks, followed by five and a half months of daily oral magnesium tablets (250 mg magnesium taurate). The remaining 8 participants, in the placebo group, were given ten placebo IVs over the next two weeks, then placebo pills for five and a half months. The volunteers in both groups treated any migraines they had with tablets containing 25 mg of sumatriptan, and kept a diary of their symptoms.

Following six months of magnesium replacement therapy, levels had risen to normal in nine of the twelve people in the magnesium group. Of those twelve, six (50 percent) now responded to sumatriptan. One other, who still had a low magnesium level, also now benefited from the drug.

In the placebo group, magnesium levels had risen to normal in two of the eight, and one of those now responded to sumatriptan. Two others, whose magnesium levels were still low, were now helped by the drug.

In sum, seven of the twelve people in the magnesium-replacement group, or 58 percent, were now able to benefit

[2] Cady RK, et al. "The effect of magnesium on the responsiveness of migraineurs to a 5-HT1 agonist." *Neurology* 50, April 1998, A340.

from sumatriptan. Only three of the eight in the placebo group, or 38 percent, responded better to the drug.

MAGNESIUM CAN ALSO HELP WITH CLUSTER HEADACHES

With all our success tying magnesium to migraines, we wondered if low magnesium levels were to blame for other types of headaches as well. We were particularly curious about cluster headaches, which typically strike men between the ages of twenty and forty. Clusters are terribly painful and come in groups: You'll often suffer from up to several per day for many days, weeks, or even months. Then they'll disappear for a while, until the next cluster or group of attacks begins. Individual cluster headaches are brief compared to migraines, usually lasting between 30 and 90 minutes, but are so intense that they're sometimes called "suicide headaches."

The cluster headache had long been considered a cousin to the migraine, and the two had been grouped together under the heading of vascular headache. Could it be that a lack of magnesium—specifically serum ionized magnesium—was the culprit in clusters? And would replacing the missing mineral relieve the pain?

My colleagues and I set about answering these questions in a study of twenty-two cluster headache patients.[3] Seven women and fifteen men, ranging in age from twenty-two to fifty, volunteered to participate. Two of them suffered from chronic cluster headaches, the other twenty from episodic clusters. We drew

[3] Mauskop A, Altura BT, Cracco RQ, Altura BM. "Intravenous magnesium sulfate relieves cluster headaches in patients with low serum ionized magnesium levels." *Headache* 1995;35:597–600.

the patients' blood to check their magnesium levels, then each was given an intravenous injection of magnesium (1 gram of $MgSO_4$). If the mineral worked—that is, if the headache was aborted and did not come back for at least two days—the patients were given another 1–2 grams of IV magnesium. The twenty-two patients received a total of thirty-nine magnesium infusions.

In fourteen of the volunteers, magnesium produced improvement that lasted at least two days and prevented at least two expected cluster attacks from striking. And in nine of them (41 percent), the relief was clinically significant. We also showed that if the serum ionized magnesium was low at the beginning of the cluster attack (a mean value of 0.521 mmol/L), patients were likely to benefit from the magnesium. But if this level was high when the cluster struck (a mean value of 0.561 mmol/L), they were not helped by the mineral.

This was not a double-blind study, which means that the placebo effect may have accounted for some of our success. (Some of the patients may have gotten better because they believed they would, rather than because the magnesium had a medicinal effect.) Despite this, we pointed to the possibility that low levels of serum ionized magnesium could be triggering cluster headaches, and that the mineral could halt attacks in progress and prevent future ones from striking.

Resources

Web Sites

The Web sites of the organizations dedicated to pain management or headaches are good places to start learning all about migraines.

The New York Headache Center—http://www.NYHeadache.com
Here, at my clinic's Web site, you'll find useful articles on migraines and other headaches, including a discussion of the types of headaches and a look at numerous medical and alternative treatments.

AAPM (The American Academy of Pain Management)—http://www.aapainmanage.org
The AAPM is the nation's largest physician-based organization dedicated to eradicating pain. At its Web site you'll find a Patient's Bill of Rights and help in finding pain-management programs. You can also read past issues of the organization's newsletter.

ACHE (American Council for Headache Education)—http://achenet.org

ACHE offers a great deal of information on women and migraines, children and headaches, and other topics, as well as links to support groups.

Headache Central—http://www.medsupport.com/survival/survival.htm

You'll find some down-to-earth advice for dealing with headaches at this site.

M.A.G.N.U.M. (Migraine Awareness Group)—http://www.migraines.org

This Web site offers interesting information on migraines, including frequently asked questions and profiles on medications.

The National Headache Foundation—http://www.Headaches.org

The foundation's Web site includes educational resources and a guide to headache types, symptoms, triggers, and therapies.

Natural Science Corporation of America—http://www.migrelief.com

This is the Web site of the company that developed MigraLief®, the patented formulation of magnesium, riboflavin, and feverfew.

Selected Bibliography

Physicians and other healthcare providers, as well as interested laypeople, can find a great deal of information about the use of magnesium, riboflavin, and feverfew in the treatment of migraines and other headaches in these articles:

Cady RK, et al. "The effect of magnesium on the responsiveness of migraineurs to a 5-HT1 agonist." *Neurology* 50, April 1998, A340.

Chia, Sin-Eng, et al. *Prevalence of Headache among Handheld Cellular Telephone Users in Singapore: A Community Study.* Department of Community, Occupational & Family Medicine, National University of Singapore, Singapore, Republic of Singapore. *Environ Health Perspect* 108:1059–62 (2000).

Durlach J, et al. "Magnesium and therapeutics." *Magnes Res* 7(3–4):313–28, 1994.

Facchinetti F, et al. "Magnesium prophylaxis of menstrual migraine: effects on intracellular magnesium." *Headache* 1991;31:298–301.

Johnson ES, Kadam NP, Hylands DM, Hylands PJ. "Efficacy of feverfew as prophylactic treatment of migraine." *Br Med J (Clin Res Ed)* 1985 Aug 31;291(6495):569–73.

Mauskop A. "Migraine Headache." In: *Neurology Practice Guidelines.* Eds. Lechtenberg and Schutta. New York: Marcel Dekker, 1997.

Mauskop A. Guest Editor. Neurobiology of Migraine. *Clinical Neuroscience* 1998; Vol. 5.

Mauskop A, Altura BM. "Magnesium for Migraine: Rationale for use and Therapeutic Potential." *CNS Drugs* 1998; 9:185–90.

Mauskop A, Altura BM. "Role of Magnesium in the Pathogenesis and Treatment of Migraines." *Clinical Neuroscience* 1998;5:24–28.

Mauskop A, Brill, MA. *The Headache Alternative: A Neurologist's Guide to Drug-Free Relief.* New York: Dell Books, 1997.

Mauskop A, Altura BT, Cracco RQ, Altura BM. "Serum ionized magnesium levels during and between migraine attacks." *Clinical Research* 40:657A, 1992. Abstract.

Mauskop A, Altura BT, Cracco RQ, Altura BM. "Serum ionized magnesium and calcium in headache classification." *Soc Neurosci Abstr* 18(1):201, 1992. Abstract.

Mauskop A, Altura BT, Cracco RQ, Altura BM. "The role of serum ionized magnesium in menstrual migraine." Proceedings of the American Pain Society's Annual Meeting, San Diego, Calif., 1992. Abstract.

Mauskop A, Altura BT, Cracco RQ, Altura BM. "Serum ionized magnesium (IMG^{2+}) in classification of patients (P) with daily headaches (DH)." Proceedings of the VIth International Headache Congress. Paris, France. August 26–29, 1993. *Cephalalgia* 1993;13:238. Abstract.

Mauskop A, Altura BT, Cracco RQ, Altura BM. "Serum ionized magnesium (IMG^{2+}) levels in patients (P) with episodic and chronic cluster headaches (CH)." *ClinPharm Ther* 53(2):227, 1993. Abstract.

Mauskop A, Altura BT, Cracco RQ, Altura BM. "Deficiency in serum ionized magnesium but not total magnesium in patients with migraines. Possible role of ICa^{2+}/IMg^{2+} ratio." *Headache* 1993;33:135–38.

Mauskop A, Altura BT, Cracco RQ, Altura BM. "Serum ionized magnesium levels in patients with tension-type headaches." In *Tension-type Headache: Classification, Mechanisms, and Treatment.* Olesen J and Schoenen J, eds. New York: Raven Press, 1993, 137–40.

Mauskop A, Altura BT, Cracco RQ, Altura BM. "Serum ionized magnesium (IMG^{2+}) levels and $ICa^{2+}/IMSP^+$ ratio as biological markers for certain headache types." Proceedings of the Fifth World Congress on Pain. Paris, France. August 22–27, 1993. Abstract.

Mauskop A, Altura BT, Cracco RQ, Altura BM. "The incidence of serum ionized magnesium deficiency in patients with an acute migraine headache is higher than in patients with an acute tension-type headache." Proceedings of the 35th Annual Scientific Meeting of the American Association for the Study of Headache, June 1993. Abstract.

Mauskop A, Altura BT, Cracco RQ, Altura BM. "Chronic daily headache—one disease or two. Diagnostic role of serum ionized magnesium." *Cephalalgia* 1994;14:24–28.

Mauskop A, Altura BT, Cracco RQ, Altura BM. "Ionized Mg, total Mg, and ICa^{2+} ratios in patients with episodic (ECH) and chronic (CCH) cluster headaches." *Headache Quarterly, Current Treatment and Research* 1994;5(2):156–58.

Mauskop A, Altura BT, Cracco RQ, Altura BM. "Serum ionized magnesium deficiency is common in women with menstrual migraine." *Neurology* 1994; 44 (4 suppl): 243S. Abstract.

Mauskop A, Altura BT, Cracco RQ, Altura BM. "Treatment of cluster headaches with intravenous magnesium sulfate." Proceedings of the 13th Annual Scientific Meeting of the American Pain Society, 1994. Abstract.

Mauskop A, Altura BT, Cracco RQ, Altura BM. "Intravenous magnesium sulfate relieves cluster headaches in patients with low serum ionized magnesium levels." *Clin Pharm Ther* 57(2):201, 1995. Abstract.

Mauskop A, Altura BT, Cracco RQ, Altura BM. "Intravenous magnesium sulfate relieves acute migraine in patients with low serum ionized magnesium levels: a pilot study." *Clinical Science* 1995;89:633–636.

Mauskop A, Altura BT, Cracco RQ, Altura BM. "Intravenous magnesium sulfate relieves cluster headaches in patients with low serum ionized magnesium levels." *Headache* 1995;35:597–600.

Mauskop A, Altura B, Cracco R, Altura B. "Intravenous magnesium sulfate rapidly alleviates headaches of various types." *Headache* 1996;36:154–60.

Mauskop A, Altura BT, Cracco RQ, Altura BM. "Serum ionized magnesium levels as a biological marker in patients with headaches." *Headache Quarterly, Current Treatment and Research* 1996;7(2):142–44.

Mauskop A, Altura BT, Cracco RQ, Altura BM. "Intravenous magnesium for the prophylaxis of menstrual migraines." *Cephalalgia* 1997;17:425.

Mauskop A, Altura BT, Cracco RQ, Altura BM. "Intravenous magnesium sulfate aborts migraine headache attacks in patients with low serum ionized magnesium levels." In *Advances in Magnesium Research: 1.* R Smetana, ed. London: John Libbey, 1997, 238–42.

Murphy JJ, Heptinstall S, Mitchell JR. "Randomised double-blind placebo-controlled trial of feverfew in migraine prevention." *Lancet* 1988 July 23;2(8604):189–92.

Peikert, A, Wilimzig C, Kohne-Volland R. "Prophylaxis of migraine with oral magnesium: results from a prospective, multi-center, placebo-controlled and double-blind randomized study." *Cephalalgia* 1996;16:257–63.

Pfaffenrath V, Wessely P, Meyer C, et al. "Magnesium in the prophylaxis of migraine—A double-blind, placebo-controlled study." *Cephalalgia* 1996;16:436–40.

Pines N, et al. "Magnesium sulphate in the treatment of angiospasm." *Lancet* 1933;1:577–79.

Pittler MH, Vogler BK, Ernst E. "Feverfew as a preventive treatment for migraine: a systematic review." *Cephalalgia* 1998;18:704–8.

Prusinski A, Durko A, Niczyporuk-Turek A. [Feverfew as a prophylactic treatment of migraine]. *Neurol Neurochir Pol* 1999;33 Suppl 5:89–95. [Article in Polish]

Schoenen J, et al. "Effectiveness of high-dose riboflavin in migraine prophylaxis. A randomized controlled trial." *Neurology* 50(2):466–70, 1998.

Schoenen J, Lenaerts M, Bastings E. "High-dose riboflavin as a prophylactic treatment of migraine: results of an open pilot study." *Cephalalgia* 1994;14:328–29.

Southon S, et al. "Micronutrient undernutrition in British schoolchildren." *Proc Nutr Soc* 52:155–63, 1993.

Wang F, Van Den Eden S, Ackerson L, Salk S, Reince R. "Oral magnesium oxide prophylaxis of frequent childhood migraine." *Cephalalgia* 2000;20:424.

Weaver K. "Magnesium and migraine." *Headache* 1990;30:168.

Index

------◀○▶------